CAROLINE CLAYTON is a journalist with a keen interest in women's health. Caroline is also the author of *Coping with Thrush*, the new edition of which was published by Sheldon Press in 1994.

Overcoming Common Problems Series

For a full list of titles please contact
Sheldon Press, Marylebone Road, London NW1 4DU

Antioxidants
DR ROBERT YOUNGSON

The Assertiveness Workbook
A plan for busy women
JOANNA GUTMANN

Beating the Comfort Trap
DR WINDY DRYDEN AND JACK
GORDON

Birth Over Thirty Five
SHEILA KITZINGER

Body Language
How to read others' thoughts by their
gestures
ALLAN PEASE

Body Language in Relationships
DAVID COHEN

Calm Down
How to cope with frustration and anger
DR PAUL HAUCK

Cancer – A Family Affair
NEVILLE SHONE

The Cancer Guide for Men
HELEN BEARE AND NEIL PRIDDY

The Candida Diet Book
KAREN BRODY

Caring for Your Elderly Parent
JULIA BURTON-JONES

Cider Vinegar
MARGARET HILLS

Comfort for Depression
JANET HORWOOD

Coping Successfully with Hayfever
DR ROBERT YOUNGSON

**Coping Successfully with Joint
Replacement**
DR TOM SMITH

Coping Successfully with Migraine
SUE DYSON

Coping Successfully with Pain
NEVILLE SHONE

Coping Successfully with Panic Attacks
SHIRLEY TRICKETT

Coping Successfully with PMS
KAREN EVENNETT

**Coping Successfully with Prostate
Problems**
ROSY REYNOLDS

**Coping Successfully with Your Hiatus
Hernia**
DR TOM SMITH

**Coping Successfully with Your Irritable
Bladder**
JENNIFER HUNT

**Coping Successfully with Your Irritable
Bowel**
ROSEMARY NICOL

Coping with Anxiety and Depression
SHIRLEY TRICKETT

Coping with Blushing
DR ROBERT EDELMANN

Coping with Breast Cancer
DR EADIE HEYDERMAN

Coping with Bronchitis and Emphysema
DR TOM SMITH

Coping with Candida
SHIRLEY TRICKETT

Coping with Chronic Fatigue
TRUDIE CHALDER

Coping with Coeliac Disease
KAREN BRODY

Coping with Cystitis
CAROLINE CLAYTON

Coping with Depression and Elation
DR PATRICK McKEON

Coping with Eczema
DR ROBERT YOUNGSON

Coping with Endometriosis
JO MEARS

Coping with Fibroids
MARY-CLAIRE MASON

Coping with Headaches
SHIRLEY TRICKETT

Coping with a Hernia
DR DAVID DELVIN

Coping with Psoriasis
PROFESSOR RONALD MARKS

Coping with Rheumatism and Arthritis
DR ROBERT YOUNGSON

Coping with Stammering
TRUDY STEWART AND JACKIE
TURNBULL

Coping with Stomach Ulcers
DR TOM SMITH

Overcoming Common Problems Series

Overcoming Common Problems Series

Overcoming Common Problems

COPING WITH CYSTITIS

Caroline Clayton

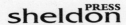

First published in Great Britain in 1995 by
Sheldon Press, SPCK, Marylebone Road, London NW1 4DU

© Caroline Clayton 1995

Third impression 2001

British Library Cataloguing-in-Publication Data
A catalogue record for this book is available from the British Library

ISBN 0–85969–715–0

Typeset by Deltatype Ltd, Ellesmere Port, Cheshire
Printed in Great Britain by
Biddles Ltd, *www.biddles.co.uk*

Contents

Acknowledgements

I would like to thank the following for their help and advice: Dr Robert Astley-Cowper, Consultant Physician/Clinic Director, Department of Genito-urinary Medicine/AIDS Unit, Northampton General Hospital NHS Trust; Karena Callen, Health and Beauty Director of *Cosmopolitan* magazine; Nancy Roberts of *Marie Claire*; Dr Jean Monroe, Medical Director of the Breakspear Hospital for Allergy and Environmental Medicine; Paul Richfield, also of the Breakspear Hospital; Sheila Ryan, RSHOM; The Women's Health Information Centre; and British Diabetic Association.

Special thanks to Alice Bulman, Kathryn Brown, Stella Cheetham, Jill Churchill, Mike Clowes, Brenda Davidson, Jacqui Deevoy, Margaret Hatton, Anne Jenkins, Julie Johnson, Tracy King, Judith Miller, Joanna Moriarty, Chris Newberry, Alison Noone, Suzie Price and Pamela Sloan, who gave me their help, encouragement and support.

Introduction

The first time I got cystitis I was meeting a friend for lunch. I went to the loo just before she arrived and immediately had to go again. She was waiting for me when I came out. 'I'm sorry,' I said, 'I don't know what's wrong but I think I'll have to go to the loo again.' 'I think you've got cystitis,' she said.

Cystitis is one of the most common and most painful everyday health problems around. In fact, cystitis is *so* common that it is very difficult to estimate exactly how many women are sufferers. Research suggests an amazing four out of five women suffer from cystitis at some time in their lives. One survey revealed that many women regard cystitis-like feelings as normal because they occur so frequently. Another survey confirmed that one in five women between the ages of 20 and 64 had experienced burning or pain on passing urine in the past year; in nearly 10 per cent of these cases, the pain had lasted for more than two weeks. But only one in ten of the sufferers had consulted her GP. Official figures, therefore, if there were any, would only serve to underestimate the extent of the problem.

During the course of my research, one thing was very noticeable: virtually every woman I spoke to about cystitis knew something about it. Those who hadn't had first-hand experience of cystitis themselves had at least some knowledge of the illness through a friend's or relation's suffering.

For most women, their first attack is the worst – simply because they do not understand what is wrong and fear the worst. That's why information is so valuable in helping prevent cystitis and pinpointing a permanent cure. In the past, many women have resigned themselves to being recurrent cystitis sufferers, believing there is little they can do about it. This is a tragedy because it needn't be the case. If you read on, you'll find out why.

1

What is cystitis?

Why cystitis can be a big pain in more ways than one

An attack always seems to come out of the blue. And as soon as it starts I remember how painful having cystitis is.

My bladder felt unusually full and I found it hard to hold on as I made my way to the loo. As I passed water the relief felt wonderful. Then, as I finished peeing, a sharp pain shot through me like a knife. 'Oh oh,' I thought, 'it's cystitis again.' I knew I was in for a sleepless night, never far from the bathroom. I started counting the hours until the doctor's surgery opened and I could get some antibiotics.

I felt bursting for the loo. But I'd been so many times that I had no urine left to pass. So I started to pass blood. That really freaked me out!

I'm always surprised how suddenly an attack can begin. One minute I'm fine, the next I'm in agony.

The burning pain is hard to bear. And the backache's a real killer.

I suddenly feel desperate for the loo and when I try to go, nothing comes out. When I realize that I've got cystitis, I get all hot and bothered and go back to the loo and try again. All that happens is a sort of drip, drip, drip instead of a huge piddle, piddle, piddle.

Ask any woman who's ever had it and she'll tell you that cystitis is a pain. It's the sort of pain you never forget – the sort of pain that floors you – and trying to cope with it can take all your time, energy and attention.

You need to go to the loo – urgently! It's difficult to pass urine and the tiny trickle that you might manage to force out comes to a finish with a big burning sensation. When you stand up to leave the bathroom, you realize that you need to go again. Your bladder feels as full as it did before. You've got cystitis.

What is cystitis?

Healthy humans aren't usually aware of their bladders. OK, if you've not been to the toilet for a while you'll eventually start to think about passing water. But then, once the deed is done, things are usually all over with for a few hours or so. With cystitis it's different. Suddenly you're aware of your bladder. It feels full and heavy and really uncomfortable – all the time.

Cystitis is an inflammation or infection of the bladder. Most cystitis sufferers have urethritis, too, which is an inflammation of the *urethra* (the tube that connects the bladder to the outside of the body). In fact, the urethra sometimes becomes inflamed first, the inflammation then spreading upwards to the bladder. Sometimes blood will be found in the urine from the inflamed urethra or bladder. Often the urine will contain pus, too, which consists of the white blood cells the body produces to fight the infection.

These symptoms are generally recognized as signs of cystitis, although not everyone with the condition suffers from the full range. Partly because it's so painful and partly because cystitis affects the very organs that affirm a woman's sexuality and feminity, cystitis can be emotionally devastating. Recurrent sufferers will need special sympathy, friends to provide an understanding ear and a patient doctor. Some doctors believe that cystitis isn't a particularly serious illness. That's because it is often treated quickly and doesn't recur. However, if left untreated, cystitis can be very serious indeed. Backache, fever and chills are signs that the infection has worked its way up to the kidneys. Repeated kidney infections, or *pyelonephritis*, could cause kidney failure. This is why it's so important to get help as soon as you can.

All cystitis is not the same

Cystitis doesn't always affect women in the same way. That's because there are actually three different types of cystitis:

- bacterial cystitis
- non-bacterial cystitis
- a mixture of the two.

Bacterial cystitis occurs when germs infect the bladder. This is usually diagnosed by means of a urine test and treated with antibiotics.

Sometimes women experience frequent or painful urination that does not seem to have a cause and no bacteria are found in the urine. They can be said to be suffering with *non-bacterial cystitis*. Non-bacterial cystitis arises when the bladder is inflamed, perhaps because it has become bruised as a result of rough sex. Women with non-bacterial cystitis describe their symptoms in the same kinds of terms as women with bacterial cystitis – typically, wanting to go to the loo a lot and pain on doing so – although it's unusual for there to be blood (*haematuria*) or pus

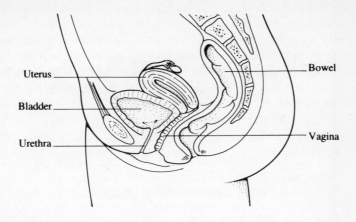

Figure 1

(*pyuria*) in the urine if no infection is present.

Some women suffer from bacterial and non-bacterial cystitis at the same time. Fortunately, having a bruised bladder and bacterial cystitis doesn't mean a double dose of pain, but your cystitis will still be very uncomfortable and you must act quickly to treat it.

A bit more about bacteria

About half, if not more, of all cystitis cases are caused by bacteria. It's thought that many tests that don't show an 'associated significant bacteriuria' (i.e. come back negative) have simply been done too early. In other words, the infection was less advanced at the time of the test and there was not enough bacteria to confirm it clinically as the main cause of the attack.

Most cases of bacterial cystitis are caused by *Escherichia coli*. *E. coli*, as it's more commonly known, is naturally present in the bowel and around your bottom, where it is quite harmless. It's only when the bacteria works its way up into the urethra and bladder that problems arise (see Figure 1).

Once inside the bladder, the bacteria multiply and irritate its lining, causing a painful inflammation. *E. coli* is particularly problematical because it can double its numbers within just half an hour. But other types of bacteria can also cause cystitis and have been found in large numbers in urine, in particular *proteus* and *Staphylococcus saprophyticus*. Proteus is often found in the intestines and staphylo*co*ccus is a germ found on the skin or mucous membranes.

Other organisms, such as *Chlamydia trachomatis* and *Candida albicans* (which causes thrush) can also inflame the urethra and cause cystitis-like sensations, but doctors regard these as very different infections. Thrush is a relatively harmless, though extremely irritating, complaint that often affects cystitis sufferers (you can read more about this in Chapter 5). Chlamydial infection is taken far more seriously by genito-urinary specialists because it can do a lot of damage if left untreated (Chlamydia is described in more detail in Chapter 14).

Sex and cystitis

Sex and cystitis enjoy a close (and painful!) relationship. Chapter 3 is devoted to describing this link and Chapter 12 details how to break it. But bacteria can affect the bladder without getting there during sex. Indeed, it's possible to get bacterial cystitis even if you've never had sex. Nuns and children, for instance, can suffer from urinary infections. Typically this happens because after a bowel movement, germs are wiped forwards from the bottom into the urethra.

> Cystitis can't be just connected with sex can it? A friend of mine had a very young baby with cystitis. Her health visitor thought the baby might have picked it up from the germs in her nappy. Now her mother is very careful to change her as often as possible and to wipe her with water and cotton wool from front to back.

> I started having cystitis when I was nine, caused by the bruising of horseriding. It felt like an intense irritation and I used to imagine that I had a horse's hair stuck in my vagina. At the time I didn't really understand that I had a frequency – I just felt irritation and soreness. It wasn't until I was 16 and started having sex that I noticed I wanted to go to the loo all the time although nothing would come out. It was really painful but I still didn't know what the matter was. I thought I must be drinking too many fluids or something. Then a year later it was diagnosed as cystitis.

About 5 per cent of young girls get cystitis before becoming sexually active. If you have a little girl, it is your responsibility as a woman to teach her to wipe herself from front to back, wiping germs *away* from the urethra towards the bottom.

Some other causes of cystitis

As we have seen, not all cystitis (whether bacterial or non-bacterial) is due to sex. There can be many other causes of an attack. Older women are more susceptible to cystitis – about a third of all women suffer their first attack after the menopause. The chemicals found in bubblebath products and vaginal deodorants can inflame the urinary tract and cause urethritis, which, for most women, feels the same as cystitis. Tampons, tea, coffee, alcohol and reactions to certain drugs can all trigger the symptoms.

> A lot of my cystitis was caused by bruising. One summer I travelled around America. I noticed if I sat down in the same position for too long I would then get cystitis and/or thrush, sitting on that particular area, being rubbed because of the movement of the bus. One time we spent three days on a Greyhound bus. I was trying to drink as much as possible, but my girlfriends thought I was greedy, drinking so much of our shared water bottle!

The very fact that cystitis/urethritis can occur as the result of so many different causes means that this condition is often talked about in fairly loose terms. Exactly how it affects sufferers also varies enormously, as the following accounts show.

> I only get cystitis if I don't go to the loo immediately after having sex. Well, not immediately but within half an hour I suppose. I have to flush away the germs. On the couple of occasions I've rolled over and gone to sleep, I've had crippling cystitis, with blood and pus and incontinence too! Drinking water and/or taking over-the-counter cystitis remedies doesn't work – antibiotics are the only cure.

> I haven't had cystitis in the same way as some of my friends have, i.e. tied to the toilet and in excruciating agony! But I've had a problem of sorts. Ever since I was a child, I've had this on/off burning pain from my bladder. It doesn't feel like I need to go to the loo, more like I haven't drunk enough. If I drink lots of water I can usually feel the burning pain subsiding. I've never mentioned it to my doctor.

> I'm lucky, when I get cystitis it only lasts two days. It usually follows an extremely active night of passion – my body's way of telling me that I've overdone things! I can cure it myself just by laying off the sex and drinking loads of water.

These and the other accounts you'll find in this book highlight the huge range of symptoms sufferers complain of. But in addition to the three main types of cystitis described here, there's also chronic cystitis – where recurrent attacks present long-term pain. And, to complicate things further, a very different type of cystitis has recently been recognized. Interstitial cystitis, as it's called, presents similar symptoms to cystitis but can actually be *caused* or *made worse* by the standard treatments for cystitis (see Chapter 15). As if this wasn't enough to contend with, there are several other infections that present the same kinds of symptoms as cystitis but are not actually cystitis. It's particularly important to know about these as some of them can cause urethritis, which in turn feels similar to an attack of cystitis! This may sound confusing, but all with be made clear.

2

A woman's problem

Why a woman's plumbing makes her prone to cystitis

Fact: cystitis is mainly a woman's problem. Women are far more susceptible to cystitis and recurrent cystitis than men. Even celibate nuns suffer with more cystitis than young sexually active men. (Kunin and McCormack)

It's simply a matter of anatomy and the differences between the male and female genitals. For a start, women have shorter urethras than men. The typical adult female's urethra is 4 cm (1½ in) long, whereas a man's is about 20 cm (8 in). Men have an added advantage in that their urethral opening is far from their anus. In women, the urethral opening is dangerously near the anus. Germs only have to travel a short distance across the perineum from the anus to reach the urethra. This is why girls should always be taught to wipe their bottoms from front to back. Wiping the other way simply brings bacteria from the bowel into areas where they can cause much harm.

The bowel is not the only threat to the urethra – the entrance to the vagina lies just a few millimetres away. Its natural secretions – a slippery acidic mucus – do not normally bother the urethra, but an infective vaginal discharge can irritate and inflame this delicate opening. There are a number of infections that affect the vagina and these are detailed in Chapter 4, save to say here that the vagina's natural acidity usually protects it against invading bacteria; it's only usually when the vagina becomes alkaline that it opens itself to infection.

Keeping the vagina healthy and yourself cystitis-free are part and parcel of the same self-help routine. Healthy sex and hygiene play a huge part in cystitis prevention (see Figure 2).

Men and cystitis

Men are less likely to suffer from cystitis than women, although they can and do get bladder infections. And they suffer from more urinary problems as they get older and their prostate glands start to play up. This gland surrounds the male urethra where it joins the bladder and, during

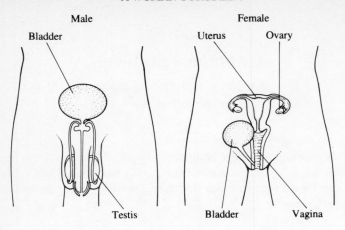

Figure 2

ejaculation, it produces a fluid that forms part of the semen. As a man ages, his prostate can become enlarged and start interfering with the outflow of urine. Although the bladder feels full, very little urine can be passed, and stagnating urine retained in the bladder may cause bacterial cystitis. Often, the only cure for prostate trouble is surgically to remove the enlarged gland.

Men and urethritis

Although so many women suffer from cystitis, pure urethritis is actually quite rare in women. Men, though, are much more likely to suffer from urethritis.

It's very easy to differentiate between urethritis and cystitis. Because men have such a long urethra, doctors can analyse urine specimens from their urethras and bladders separately, using the 'two glass test'. For this, the man will be asked to pass a small amount of urine into one glass (this is the urine passed from the urethra) and then the rest into another glass (this will be the urine from the bladder). Doctors diagnose urethritis if the urine in the first glass contains small 'casts' (these look just like threads) and the urine in the second glass is crystal clear urine. It's only likely that the man has true cystitis (a bladder infection) if the urine in the second glass is cloudy or contains protein.

Male urethritis is typically caused by a host of organisms, almost all of which are acquired sexually. Therefore, it is often referred to as non-specific urethritis (NSU) until the bacteria causing the infection (e.g.

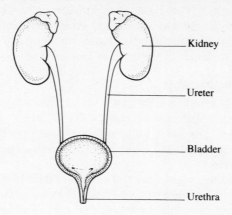

Kidney

Ureter

Bladder

Urethra

Figure 3

chlamydia or gonorrhoea) can be identified. Many cases of NSU remain unexplained but, for both men and women, prevention is better than cure.

How the urinary system works

You don't have to be a doctor to understand what cystitis is and how best to beat it. However, the urinary system – the body's way of filtering out and disposing of waste – is pretty complicated. For most people, most of the time, this system ticks over very nicely without causing any problems, but things can and do go wrong. Often knowing *why* something has happened is the first step towards making sure it doesn't happen again. So, let us look at how the urinary system works.

The kidneys

Urine starts its journey in the kidneys, which are two bean-shaped organs that filter the blood to remove waste materials from it. These complicated precision instruments are very robust and don't succumb to disease easily. When one kidney fails, the other simply doubles up its workload. But if both fail, then you're in trouble. Kidney disease is very serious because waste products build up in the body, poisoning it (see Figure 3).

On average, the kidneys filter about 170 litres (360 pints) of fluid every day – that's about a thousand cups of tea! Almost all of this filtered material is reabsorbed into the bloodstream. Only waste products are separated out to be excreted along with any excess salts and about 1 to 1.7

litres (2 to 3 pints) of water. This is the amount of fluid normally excreted in a day. This fluid flows down from each kidney to the bladder via long tubes called ureters (not to be confused with the ureth*ra*). Each tube has a valve at the end. Pressure mounts as urine builds up in the ureters and this opens the valve, allowing the urine to pass into the bladder.

The bladder and urethra

The bladder is a bit like a balloon – round when it's full and flat when empty. The adult bladder holds about 400 to 500 ml ($\frac{3}{4}$ pint) of urine. Its walls expand as it begins to fill up with the fluids from the kidneys. Once the bladder is about half full, nerve fibres in its walls signal to the brain that it needs emptying.

Normal, healthy adults have full control of their bladders and urethral reflexes, which they learn when they are very young. This control centres around contracting a voluntary sphincter – the circular layer of muscle surrounding the urethra. This keeps the urethra closed despite strong bladder contractions. Learning to control urination helps us to progress from helpless toddlers into independent people. By temporarily suppressing the bladder's contractions, we can ignore the urge to urinate until it is convenient to go. This ability to exercise mind over matter certainly makes life easier, but this control should never be abused. The more the bladder fills up, the more it must stretch. The longer you leave going to the toilet, the greater the pressure you put on your bladder. Anyone who suffers from cystitis should make a habit of emptying their bladder as soon as possible after first feeling the urge to do so.

Because the root of cystitis often lies in the bladder, this organ has been the subject of much research. Doctors have been puzzled as to why patients only develop bacterial cystitis at certain times as bacteria can find a way into the urethra and bladder almost all the time. A healthy urethra and bladder *can* withstand an invasion of bacteria, but only up to a point. Normal urine is acidic, so it's hostile to germs – a crucial factor in the fight against cystitis. The bladder's best defence, however, is to empty itself regularly. This way, germs are flushed out of the body before they can build up and cause an infection. This is why women who are susceptible to cystitis should drink plenty of fluids and go to the toilet as often as possible. Frequent urination is the key to keeping bacteria in the bladder at a harmless level. Urine allowed to stagnate in the bladder becomes a breeding ground for bacteria. Women and men who are unable to empty their bladders fully often develop infections.

Recurrent cystitis has also intrigued doctors, and much research has been done to try and discover what it is that makes a woman prone to repeated infections. Again, scientists looked at the bladder in search of an answer and, more specifically, the cells in the bladder wall. Research by J. Fowler and T. A. Stamey suggests that bacterial cystitis temporarily changes the surface of the urethra and bladder and makes them immediately more attractive to bacteria. In other words, the more you suffer from bacterial cystitis, the more difficult it becomes to resist further attacks. Fowler and Stamey's research suggests that cells on the inner lining change after the first attack of cystitis and alien bacteria find it easier to adhere to them. If you're suffering from your second attack or more in the last few months, please don't panic though – you can compensate for a lowered resistance to urinary tract infections. Keep drinking, keep going to the toilet and read on!

3

Cystitis and sex

When bacteria and bruising spell
double trouble

My cystitis has almost always been triggered by sexual activity of a 'rewarding kind'! Hence the double frustration, conflict and paradox!

My cystitis is brought on by intercourse. The trouble is that for me sex always feels better, more pleasurable, on a full bladder. Maybe that's why I'm more prone to it.

If you've had sex within the 48 hours prior to the beginning of an attack, you'd be right in thinking that the sex and cystitis were closely related.

Sex very often causes cystitis. That's because sex can push bacteria into the urethra and bladder, causing an infection to arise. On the other hand, some doctors see so many cases of non-bacterial cystitis triggered by intercourse that they often refer to it as sexual cystitis – the bladder and urethra become bruised and inflamed and present the same sorts of symptoms as a urinary infection.

Bacteria and sex

As mentioned before, about half of all cystitis cases are caused by bacteria and, unfortunately, there's nothing better than sex for pushing a few germs into places they shouldn't be. Our bodies naturally harbour many different kinds of bacteria, often without causing problems. It's only when they stray into areas they shouldn't that they cause difficulties. Cystitis, for example, can start when bacteria naturally present around the anus work their way into the urethra.

It's common and perfectly natural for bacteria to enter the urethra during sex. Interestingly, some women don't seem to be affected by the presence of these bacteria in their urethras. They can harbour these germs for a while without any harmful effects. For the rest of us, though, urinating immediately after sex will flush the bacteria out of the bladder and urethra so they can do no harm. It also makes sense for any sexually active woman to wash before sex, practise good vaginal hygiene generally and always wipe from front to back! Studies have shown that the urethra of a woman with recurrent urinary tract infections tends to be invaded by *E. coli* rather than any other organism. This germ is the major cause of bacterial cystitis. By generally waging war against *E. coli*, therefore, you reduce your chances of succumbing to cystitis.

Because the vaginal, anal and urethral openings are so close, bacteria can very easily travel from one opening to another during sexual activity. Anything that comes into contact with the anus should be washed before it touches the urethral area, to prevent the spread of *E. coli*.

> I've had cystitis three times and it's always been brought on by the same thing – having anal sex and vaginal sex, one after the other without washing! It's hard to think about hygiene when you're doing things like that!

> I dread to think where I'd be today if I hadn't read about the cystitis–sex connection. Nobody told me that having sex could give you cystitis. Once I learned to pass water within 15 minutes of having sex I said goodbye to suffering.

> I suppose the semen irritated my urethra and caused the attacks. If you think about it, semen is a foreign body – your body reacts to it in the same way that it would react to any strange organism.

Non-bacterial cystitis and its causes

If you thought the link between sex and cystitis was just bacteria, think again. Having sex can cause a non-bacterial type of cystitis/urethritis, too. Even the most scrupulously clean women who wash and urinate before and after sex without fail can find themselves prone to attacks. The main reason for this is down to a woman's plumbing again! A woman's bladder and urethra lie just in front of her vagina. Any object inserted into a woman's vagina and moved up and down will rub against the bladder through the vaginal wall. Rough, vigorous sex can therefore trigger off an attack of cystitis because the urethra and bladder become bruised, inflamed, sensitive and sore.

> After sex my bladder feels bruised. Urinating doesn't sting but it just doesn't feel right. I'm aware of my bladder like it's telling me it's there! The sensation wears off after a couple of days or so . . . but at the time it's painful enough to rule out sex for a while.

Cystitis sufferers may find that some sexual positions irritate the bladder and urethra more than others. And these can differ depending on the partner. There's more about this in Chapter 12, but the best advice for anyone prone to recurrent attacks is to take it easy.

Cystitis and sex – the facts

Doctors have spent time researching which acts of sex are more likely to cause cystitis than others because, as you may know yourself, even sex in the most adventurous positions doesn't automatically bring on an attack. What they have found is that women are most at risk when they have a burst of sexual activity after not having had intercourse for a while.

> Sometimes my partner and I go through periods when we make love a lot. When we don't have sex for a few weeks – which sometimes happens if we're working hard or he's travelling – it takes my body a while to get used to it again. It's like the more we do it, the more comfortable it is and the less sore I feel afterwards.

Cystitis used to be known as the honeymoon disease because often the very first act of intercourse a woman had would leave her toilet-tied and in pain.

> Losing my virginity was a fantastic experience. I felt so happy and warm about it. Unfortunately, I soon had the smile wiped off my face. Forty-eight hours later I got cystitis. I'd never had it before; I was in a terrible state. I thought I must have caught a horrible disease from my man. Looking back on it now I think the pain I went through spoilt the whole sexual experience for me.

> I almost always get cystitis or thrush after sleeping with a new boyfriend. It's as if my body is really anti having any alien saliva or sperm anywhere near me!

Women also seem to be more prone to sexual cystitis if they have sex often in a short space of time. This stands to reason. If the sensitive tissues of the bladder and urethra are bruised, they will need time to heal. Otherwise, tiny cracks in the injured tissues can become a breeding ground for bacteria, which may ultimately work their way into the bladder. So, sex can trigger both bacterial and non-bacterial cystitis at the same time. And if you've ever suffered from both you'll probably agree that sex can indeed be a double-edged sword!

> For me, cystitis seems to go hand in hand with sex. I spent six months in Japan away from my boyfriend. During this six months when I didn't have sex, my previously painful cystitis completely disappeared.

> I had a serious relationship in my early twenties and cystitis became an almost continual problem. I was getting kidney infections a lot, too,

16

and it got to the point when I couldn't bear to have sex because I was so scared of getting cystitis. I'd clamp up during sex. My boyfriend thought I was frigid and said I should have sex counselling. All the problems of our relationship were being dumped on my cystitis.

Cystitis can make sex painful and distressing; it can even ruin a relationship altogether.

Some women find their sexual cystitis disappears without treatment from a doctor. They find that they can calm down the symptoms of cystitis by drinking plenty of plain water until the bruised tissues have healed themselves, or that if they follow a detailed self-help plan (as outlined in Chapter 12) they can avoid having attacks after intercourse. But anyone who suffers from repeated attacks would be wise to do some detective work to identify other possible triggers. Chapter 4 describes what these are.

4

What else can cause cystitis?

If you've already flicked through this book to the diagnostic chart in Chapter 17, you'll realize that cystitis can have a multiplicity of causes. One of the problems facing women today is that there are just so many possible triggers of an attack of cystitis that it's hard to know where to begin looking for the culprit. So let's take a look at what researchers have discovered.

When you've gotta go, you've gotta go!

One survey (Adatto, et al.) found that the biggest single factor in predisposing women to cystitis was putting off passing urine for an hour or more. A group of young women who suffered from recurrent urinary infections were compared with a control group. The purpose of the control group was to give the doctors an insight into the urination habits of women who had never had cystitis and, interestingly, almost 90 per cent of these women emptied their bladders regularly and completely. On the other hand, two thirds of the cystitis sufferers admitted to regularly putting off a trip to the toilet, sometimes for more than six hours after they first had the urge to go! Most of the cystitis sufferers admitted to putting off going for more than three hours, which appeared to be something they had done since they were children.

Strangely enough, there was actually very little difference in the total number of times the women went to the toilet in any one day. What the cystitis-prone group appeared to be doing was avoiding urinating during the day and making up for this in their own homes at night – to the detriment of their health. The reasons given for delaying visits to the toilet were 'embarrassment in social situations' and 'an unwillingness to use public toilets or interrupt activities in which they were engaged'.

I was working in a busy department. I seemed to spend my days rushing around. There always seemed to be someone who wanted me, someone I had to speak to and organize. I'd often find myself desperate for the loo, but I'd almost always ignore the urge. I soon became quite constipated and developed cystitis too. I realized I'd better make time for myself and the most important functions of the day!

All the women studied were asked about their sexual habits and their hygiene routines too. No noticeable differences were found so this survey strongly points to putting off urination as the biggest single cause of recurrent cystitis.

Let's look at why this should be so. When the bladder is full, it becomes distended and less able to resist infection by bacteria naturally present in the intestine. So holding on damages the bladder. Another survey (Cox and Hinman) proved that emptying the bladder frequently actually helps reduce the likelihood of getting cystitis and other urinary tract infections. This is because bacteria are flushed away before they can build up their numbers to harmful levels. Also, emptying the bladder within ten minutes of having sexual intercourse is an essential part of preventing cystitis.

Tampons, bacteria and bladder infections

One survey searching for a common link in women suffering from recurrent urinary tract infections was conducted at UCLA's School of Public Health, USA. It looked at risk factors, such as diet, clothing and urination habits. This research found another two strong candidates to blame: tampons and soft drinks. Many of the women suffering from cystitis (either for the first time or who had recurrent attack) reported using tampons. It's not known exactly *how* using tampons can trigger cystitis, but it's believed that they may help spread bacteria from the vagina to the urethral opening. Inserted tampons might also press against the urethra, preventing complete emptying of the bladder.

Tampons made from bleached cotton fibre may cause allergy-related cystitis. Many women are also sensitive to the chemicals found in superabsorbant or deodorized tampons and sanitary towels.

Superslim, superabsorbant towels contain chemicals such as *polyacrylate gels* (also found in disposable nappies), which can absorb many times their own weight in liquid. These gels can irritate delicate skin (if they are inhaled they can cause lung problems). Chemically impregnated towels, tampons and panty liners can irritate the delicate mucous membranes of the vagina. The first rule of women's health is: *never put anything inside your vagina that you wouldn't put into your mouth*.

If you must use tampons, look for unbleached cotton or chlorine-free ones (the ones without an applicator are kinder to the environment). And avoid tampons that have plastic applicators. These have sharp, pointed teeth, which can nick or cut the delicate skin in or around the vagina and so allow an infection to start. Wash your hands before and after inserting a tampon. To avoid the spread of bacteria, remember to remove your tampon with the hand you won't be using to insert its replacement.

Change your tampons every two to four hours. And use chlorine-free towels at night.

Tights and tight trousers

Doctors talk about not restricting the flow of air around your fanny! But restricting clothes can cause cystitis too. Leggings don't bother me but jeans seem to restrict me. When you sit down in jeans your whole body seems to be crushed up in them. As well as the thick seam of jeans rubbing you, the material is so stiff that they hold your pelvis in a certain unnatural way. And the way they restrict your body's natural movement can cause pressure, which in turn can cause cystitis or a cystitis-like sensation. That's why I always wear my Marks and Spencers, size 16–18, big pants! Like the old 1960s bikinis, they can't ride up between your legs. 'Bodies' are really uncomfortable too – I don't understand why women bother with them.

The wearing of tights, nylon pants and layers of tight clothing has long been blamed for causing cystitis attacks. Nylon underwear and tights, and tight jeans or trousers encourage harmful organisms, such as *E. coli* and *Candida albicans*, to multiply to nuisance levels, causing urethritis/cystitis. But the American lifestyle survey mentioned above, which tried to pinpoint causes of cystitis in young women, found only a slight risk of cystitis associated with wearing tights. This may be because more women wear opaque cotton and Lycra tights or tights with cotton gussets. Cotton absorbs sweat and vaginal moisture and air can circulate through the porous fabric, killing bacteria before they can become a problem.

There's lots more about thrush in the next chapter, but if you suspect that your cystitis is made worse by wearing tights, throw they away – now! Wear stockings or suspender tights, with an open gusset, instead. Good department stores may stock these but they are also available from some mail-order catalogues, such as Innovations (they also have several shops in the UK; see the Useful addresses section at the back of this book for their address).

Allergies and irritants

The vagina is sensitive. The delicate mucous membranes lining it tear easily and can be affected by external factors. And, as mentioned before, urethritis, which feels rather like cystitis, can also be brought on by *irritants* to the urethra and bladder. These include bath additives, vaginal deodorants, vaginal douches or the antioxidants in the rubber of condoms and caps. Some people find they are sensitive to toiletries such as vaginal deodorants, soap and/or talcum powder – that using these products causes an allergic reaction.

About 20 per cent of the general population are allergic, suffering a mild to violent reaction to substances that don't apparently affect the rest of the population. There are more and more cases of asthma, hay fever and eczema, a development that seems to be linked to the increasing pollution of food, water and air. In fact, since the 1950s, the prevalence of hypersensitivity to certain foreign substances or antigens has approximately doubled every ten years.

Most people are familiar with the 'traditional' allergies, such as hay fever – allergic rhinitis and conjunctivitis, that's when your nose streams and your eyes sting! – asthma, and rashes, such as eczema and urticaria. But, very few people associate bacterial cystitis and bladder pain with a reaction to food or environmental factors. Yet Dr Jean Monroe, Medical Director of the Breakspear Hospital for Allergy and Environmental Medicine in Hertfordshire, sees about 50 patients a year with sensitivity-related cystitis. She explains:

> The causes are almost invariably multifactorial and our treatment treats many sensitivities in each patient. Food and environmental chemicals are the most common causes of allergic cystitis, but the problem is exacerbated by new fabrics, deodorants and sanitary towels. Approximately five to ten per cent of women will experience sensitivity-related cystitis in their lifetime.

And it's not just women who are affected either: 'Men often complain of urinary symptoms similar to cystitis,' says Dr Monroe.

Recurrent cystitis and bladder pain frequently respond to a wide-ranging allergy investigation, but this has to be done by an expert. The substances causing the sensitivities must be isolated and then avoided. Unfortunately, food allergies are often reactions to favourite foods – we are usually addicted to substances we are allergic to. Of course, it's not always possible to avoid substances we are sensitive to. For example, patients living in big cities have little choice but to carry on breathing in polluted air. In cases like this the allergy can be relieved with medication or treated. Sometimes the patient can be desensitized to increase their tolerance of the substances they react most badly to.

If you've had recurrent attacks of 'unexplained' cystitis for some time, it may be that you have become sensitive to something that previously didn't bother you. Allergies aren't just inherited from a family member. They can be triggered by a virus infection, massive exposure to chemicals or radiation, or a shock or accident. The only way to know for certain if you have an allergy is to be tested. Ask your GP to refer you to a specialist in allergies and/or environmental medicine.

Pregnancy and childbirth

I've only really had cystitis since I had my baby boy. In the past I've occasionally had twinges when I felt like I desperately needed to pass water even though I'd just urinated. But this sensation would usually disappear quite quickly.

Whenever I drink while I'm eating I always get this feeling of needing to urinate a lot – it's very strange! About 15 minutes after a meal I find I can't stop going to the loo. So the first time I got cystitis I thought it was that. Then it started to hurt and although it felt like I badly needed to urinate again I could only manage to squeeze a drop out. I realized I must have cystitis as I'd read a bit about it. And since then, unfortunately, I've had cystitis quite a lot.

Cystitis is quite a common problem during pregnancy and after childbirth, due to the hormonal changes that occur. For example, the hormones released during pregnancy relax the muscle tone of the urinary system. This can lead to stress incontinence (when a small amount of urine leaks out whenever you laugh, cough or sneeze), but more worryingly, can also cause urine to be retained in the ureters and bladder. The growing baby pressing against the bladder may also prevent it from being emptied properly (large ovarian cysts or fibroids can decrease bladder capacity in the same way). Instead of being flushed out of the body as normal, bacteria in the urine start to multiply out of all proportion, inflaming the urinary tract.

Pregnant women are also more susceptible to cystitis as their kidneys have to work harder, circulating an increased amount of fluid around the body. The extra stress of this makes the urinary system more vulnerable to infection. Women with a history of cystitis or those with sickle-cell anaemia or diabetes are particularly prone to cystitis during pregnancy. If any of these apply to you, inform your pre-natal care provider.

Studies have shown that women who contract cystitis during pregnancy may have an increased risk of going into premature labour. If you have cystitis and you think there's even a possibility that you may be pregnant, tell your doctor. And always ask your GP about any antibiotics or other treatments you are prescribed – make sure they don't affect your unborn child.

Prolaspes

A survey by C. M. Kumin and R. C. McCormack found that the more times a woman gives birth, the greater her chances of suffering from cystitis. This may well be due to the fact that childbirth and pregnancy, as well as age, weaken the pelvic floor muscles, sometimes causing the uterus to drop down (prolapse). A prolapsed uterus puts pressure on the bladder wall, which may give rise to feeling the need to go to the toilet frequently.

> My cure for cystitis is abstinence from penetrative sex. I'm 75 and I'm told I have a cystocele (my bladder has prolapsed into my vagina). After 20 years of spasmodic attacks of cystitis, treated with antibiotics, I decided that there could be a correlation between the two. My husband agreed to try this method and, since then, I've had no further attacks. That was nearly 20 years ago.

To prevent urinary problems after childbirth, you must strengthen your pelvic floor muscles with special exercises. Suspension surgery can correct a prolapsed womb, but may lead to other urinary problems (see Janine's story in Chapter 16). Exercising the pelvic floor muscles before, during and after pregnancy will prevent a prolapse happening in the first place or improve the situation if you have prolapsed. In fact, it's a good idea for anyone suffering from cystitis to do these exercises daily as they will improve pelvic muscle tone, increase the circulation of blood in the pelvic area and promote healing.

All about pelvic floor muscles

The pelvic floor muscles hold all the pelvic organs in place. You can check how strong they are by starting and stopping the flow of urine when you're on the toilet. If you can do this easily, it's a good sign that these muscles are working well.

Whenever you squeeze your pelvic floor muscles, you're exercising them, which helps to keep them toned and healthy. But lots of women aren't even aware of these muscles until they give birth and attend a post-natal exercise group. All new mums should start exercising these muscles immediately and there are several ways of doing this. Starting and stopping your flow of urine is not one of them, however, as it may actually cause cystitis. Don't do it!

Instead, put aside about ten minutes each day when you can relax undisturbed. Become aware of your pelvic floor by tightening the muscles a few times. Imagine your pelvic floor as a lift that must travel up four floors. Then breathe in and draw the muscles up a little to reach the 'first floor'. Hold for a few seconds, then pull them up further to reach the 'second floor' and so on. When you've reached the 'top floor' breathe out and in once, then gradually release the muscles as you breathe out again. This is easier if you imagine the lift descending through four floors. Then repeat these exercises at least five times in a row.

You can do simpler pelvic floor exercises at any time of the day by simply squeezing then releasing the muscles. Contract the muscles hard for a few seconds, and then release them completely. Try to do this 20 times on the trot, at least five times a day. This may seem excessive, but you'll find they can be done any place, any time – you can do them while driving a car if necessary! And if you do them every day you should notice a big difference after just a few weeks.

Vaginal cones are an alternative to pelvic floor exercises. These come in several different weights. At first women use the lightest one, keeping it in the vagina for 15 minutes twice daily. As the muscles gradually strengthen, you can progress to the heavier cones. One survey compared the success rates of cones with those of Kegel pelvic floor muscle exercises and reported that 'vaginal cones were easier to teach, had a lower drop-out rate, and showed an initial advantage in strengthening the pelvic floor compared to Kegel exercises' (Norton and Baker). And a similar survey found that 'training with vaginal cones produced significantly better pelvic floor strength than did exercise without cones' (Jonasson, et al.). For, more about vaginal cones, see Chapter 14.

The menopause and cystitis

Menopause literally means 'the cessation of menstruation', but the term is used to describe the span of time covering when a woman's body starts changing and adjusting to when there are no more periods. The changes usually start to happen well before menstruation actually stops altogether.

The end of periods and no longer having to use contraception comes as a relief to many women. But the hormone shifts that accompany and follow the menopause can trigger bladder infections. Because the body then receives less oestrogen, post-menopausal women tend to have weakened urethral and vaginal walls. The lack of oestrogen also causes the urethra and the vagina to become shorter (constricted), drier and less elastic. This means they are more susceptible to bruising during intercourse which could lead to urethritis/cystitis.

I wondered whether my cystitis could be linked to my hysterectomy. A friend of mine who's a nurse told me that after this operation I'd never have the same bladder tone as I'd had before. I think that's because when they operate, they knock it about a bit. My ovaries were removed as well as my womb, which has caused other problems. My vagina is much drier than it used to be and I think this has left me with a tendency to get cystitis.

Hormone replacement therapy (or HRT as it is commonly known) is the best cure for this type of cystitis. Treatments usually contain oestrogen rather than oestrogen *and* progesterone. And they should be given in short courses in the form of vaginal creams or tablets, injections, implants or skin patches. After the first four to six weeks of oestrogen treatment, most menopausal women only need tiny top-up doses for short periods.

Sadly, it's not just cystitis that affects post-menopausal women. At this point in life you become more susceptible to vaginal infections, partly because the skin lining the vagina becomes thinner and more fragile, but also because the vagina becomes more alkaline and less able to keep potentially harmful germs in check. Fortunately, these symptoms also respond well to treatment with oestrogen.

Catheters

I've had a lot of problems with cystitis since my baby was born. Straight after the birth I tried to go to the loo but I couldn't. The nurses put a catheter in me and I wonder if that's made me more susceptible to cystitis.

If you go into hospital for an operation, you may have a catheter (a fine tube) inserted into your urethra. This is to draw off any urine that gathers in the bladder while you are unconscious and/or unable to empty your bladder yourself. But wherever possible, women prone to cystitis should avoid having catheters inserted as they can actually implant bacteria in the bladder, especially if they are in place for a long time.

Amazingly, half of all infections caught by patients in hospital are urinary tract infections, mostly caused by the use of catheters. Catheters can irritate the urethra by damaging the surface layer of cells of the urethral lining. This lining is the urethra's main defence against the invasion of bacteria. Once damaged, the urethra is open to infection. To prevent the onset of cystitis, patients are often given antibiotics after catheterization.

Theoretically speaking, it's quite easy to determine whether or not a urinary tract infection has been caused by the use of a catheter. The infecting bacteria in these cases include the germs enterobacter, proteus and/or enterococci as opposed to the more common *E. coli*.

If you have to go into hospital and you have to use a catheter, make sure it's only fitted for as short a time as necessary. Drink plenty of fluids to flush out any dangerous bacteria and make sure you urinate as soon as the catheter is removed.

The side-effect of medication

Cystitis is occasionally a side-effect of taking prescribed drugs. One such drug is tiaprofenic acid, a non-steroid anti-inflammatory drug commonly prescribed for osteoarthritis. Other drugs found to throw up cystitis as a side-effect include danazol (a drug also known as Danol, prescribed to treat endometriosis), which causes cystitis with bleeding, and an antiallergenic drug called Tranilast.

Drug related cystitis is easy to cure. Once the medication is stopped, the cystitis should disappear. But it's much better to avoid it occurring in the first place. Always ask your GP to tell you of any side-effects a drug may have before accepting a prescription.

What if no cause can be found?

It's important to remember that while some things alone may only have a slight association with cystitis, several of them together could well bring on an attack, especially if you're having sex a lot and using a diaphragm as well. Such combinations make the 'overload' factor – as the risk factors build up, you get closer to your 'cystitis threshold'.

Sometimes no apparent cause can be found at all for recurrent cystitis, and sufferers have to find a way to cope with the problem. This can be emotionally draining, so if you find yourself in this situation, you should find someone to support you. Regular physical exercise or a weekly relaxation class or massage may help you to cope better. It's important to stay healthy mentally because bladder problems are often linked with the emotions. In fact, the lower your emotional state, the more prone you are to cystitis – ironic when you consider how low cystitis can make you feel anyway!

My partner left me soon after the birth of my baby. Most of the time I managed because I wasn't used to much support from him anyway. I recovered from the birth quite quickly, but my pelvic floor was in a bit of a state. I just couldn't hold my bladder like I used to. When I did my exercises I'd notice a slight improvement. But there were times when I'd feel very angry with my ex-partner. And my bladder control was always much worse at times like these.

WHAT ELSE CAN CAUSE CYSTITIS?

The first step towards coping with cystitis is to take control of your health. It's essential to find out as much as you possibly can about the subject. With patience and persistence you will eventually seek out the underlying cause of your problem. So read on.

5

Thrush and cystitis

I don't have the classic symptoms of thrush when I get it. Instead of feeling itchy, I get a burning pain in my urethra. It doesn't hurt when I go to the toilet but it stings afterwards. And I get a dull ache in my lower back. When I first felt like this I went to my doctor but, after testing my urine, he couldn't find anything wrong with me.

It was only after talking to a friend that I realized I'd got thrush and that this was the cause of my 'cystitis-like' problems.

The thrush/cystitis cycle

Thrush and cystitis tend to occur together, but in fact thrush rarely causes *true* cystitis. Instead, it's much more likely that the thick, curdy discharge associated with thrush irritates the urethra, causing urethritis. Once the thrush has been treated, the apparent cystitis should disappear too. It sounds straightforward and, in theory, it is. The only problem is that thrush has a nasty habit of recurring, sometimes only days after you think you've got rid of it.

What is thrush and how is it caused?

Thrush is a fungal infection, caused by a yeast-like organism known as *Candida albicans*. Small numbers of the organism are naturally present in the vagina and bowel, along with many other bacteria and fungi, and in these small numbers they rarely cause a problem. The acidity of the vagina usually prevents candida, and other potentially harmful organisms, from multiplying, but, when the vagina becomes alkaline, the numbers increase and infections can occur.

Thrush is, therefore, an overgrowth of candida in the vagina. Because it thrives in warm, wet places, it's possible to get thrush in your mouth too, though this is more common in young babies than adults. The vagina offers ideal conditions in which thrush can grow, making women particularly prone to yeast infections. The surest signs of thrush are a thick, white discharge that itches like crazy! But there are many women who don't realize they have thrush until tests diagnose the infection or until they suffer from a related condition, such as cystitis.

Candida – the whole picture

It's now believed that although thrush itself isn't a serious disease, left unchecked it can cause problems. A candida overgrowth in the intestines can damage the mucus-covered lining there and lead to *leaky gut syndrome*. Put simply this means that instead of being passed out of the body, as normally happens, harmful toxic organisms in the bowel become reabsorbed into the digestive system, causing a whole range of symptoms to develop, from headaches, dizziness and nausea to acne or food allergies. And chronic candida throughout the body may cause more serious conditions, such as asthma and psoriasis.

Scientists have also drawn a link between thrush and PMT. A recent study analysing women suffering from both PMT and thrush discovered that two thirds of the women's PMT improved when their thrush was treated with antifungal drugs and diet. PMT may just be a symptom of too much candida in the body, so PMT sufferers with a history of vaginal thrush will probably be helped by an anti-candida programme too.

Extreme cases of candidiasis have been linked with ME. This is thought to be a viral condition, although some doctors don't recognize the illness. ME used to be called 'Yuppy Flu', mainly because the sufferers whose case histories were highlighted in the media tended to be high achievers with stressful lives. But this classification was misleading as ME affects a broad range of people from all walks of life. Interestingly, the symptoms ME sufferers complain of are also experienced by sufferers of chronic thrush, namely extreme fatigue, depression, lack of concentration and poor memory. And in fact, when given treatment for candida through drugs and diet, ME sufferers' symptoms have often disappeared!

Why thrush causes cystitis-like symptoms

Thrush often causes cystitis-like symptoms in women (apparent cystitis). That's because the discharge associated with the candida can irritate and inflame the urethra. And when thrush affects the urethra, it can make urinating very painful indeed. Not surprisingly then, if you are suffering from thrush you may think you have an attack of cystitis because the main symptom of cystitis is pain on passing urine.

The fact that women have relatively short urethras makes it harder to differentiate between urethritis and cystitis. In other words, if you have cystitis-like symptoms, it's difficult to know whether the pain is actually coming from the bladder or just the tube that carries urine from the bladder to the urethral opening. That's why thrush sufferers often feel like they are developing an attack of cystitis, despite the fact that their *bladders* are not inflamed.

Because so many women can't tell any difference between the symptoms of urethritis and those of cystitis, they often report to their GP with yet another attack of 'unexplained cystitis'. And even though a urine test may prove negative, showing that no offending bacteria are present, it's not uncommon for a GP to prescribe antibiotics to 'cure' their patient's symptoms. But the *worst* possible treatment in this case is antibiotics. That's because one of the side-effects of antibiotics is that they can cause an overgrowth of candida throughout the body – in effect, antibiotics can actually cause thrush or make an existing attack more severe, which further irritates the urethra. And so the cycle repeats itself.

Breaking the cycle – getting rid of thrush

The only way to treat thrush-related cystitis is to cure the root of the problem – the candida itself. For years doctors doled out local treatments for vaginal thrush – pessaries and creams that were messy, but seemed to work. For a while. After a short respite, many sufferers found that their thrush came back with a vengeance. Tests have proved that vaginal and oral thrush are only symptoms of a general overgrowth of candida throughout the body. One study examined 98 women who complained of recurrent vaginal thrush. Swabs from both the vagina and bowel were taken from each of the women. These were then compared and it was found that thrush was *always* present in the bowel if it was found in the vagina. Those who tested negative for thrush in the bowel, *never* showed candida in the vagina. It's now recognized that the only way to get rid of thrush properly and to avoid recurrent attacks – to break the thrush/cystitis cycle – is to treat the body as a whole. That means asking your doctor for an oral thrush drug and adopting an anti-candida diet and lifestyle.

Pessaries and creams

You can buy vaginal pessaries and creams for thrush from your local chemist, but these only treat the problem locally. They can't cure an overall candida problem. That's why it's important to visit your GP when you've got thrush.

A lot of women find that pessaries and creams provide relief from their symptoms. They can and do work well and the body can sometimes fight back against an overgrowth of candida, restoring its natural balance without further treatment. But very often it can't. What happens is that, after a short while, the overgrowth of candida throughout the body triggers off yet another attack of thrush.

Many women have resigned themselves to being recurrent thrush sufferers and yet this needn't be the case. It's likely that anyone who suffers from two or more attacks in a short space of time has an overall thrush infection that needs further treatment.

Oral thrush tablets

As candida in the bowel or the intestine is almost always the cause of recurrent thrush attacks, oral tablets, which work by killing off all fungi within the body, are the most effective way to clear up thrush for good. It's been proved that patients with recurrent vaginal thrush are more likely to be cured when they are treated at the same time for intestinal candidiasis.

Essentially, if you have vaginal thrush it's almost certain that other areas of your body will be infected too, though you may not realize it. So, when you take your first course of vaginal pessaries, suggest to your doctor that you take some treatment by mouth too. Oral antifungal drugs include Nystan, Nizoral, Sporanox and Diflucan. The last three are all relatively new on the market and have been developed because research has shown that women prefer to take an oral treatment rather than mess about with pessaries and creams.

Nizoral contains the drug ketoconazole, an antifungal antibiotic. When Nizoral was introduced, it seemed as if a major breakthrough in the treatment of thrush had been made. It was, and still is, claimed that Nizoral could clear up candida without the help of pessaries or creams. The same now goes for Sporanox and Diflucan, the latter being just a one-off dose and thus particularly popular with patients.

One of the main reasons women find recurrent thrush so difficult to cope with is that pessaries are messy and inconvenient to use. One discharge – the one associated with the thrush – is replaced by another – the leakage from the pessaries. In this respect, oral tablets have a distinct advantage over pessaries. Like all oral medications, however, they can have side-effects. Reported adverse effects of these types of drugs include nausea, stomach upsets and heartburn, headaches and dizziness. They shouldn't be taken by any woman who's pregnant or even thinking about becoming pregnant. If in doubt, ask your doctor's advice.

No sex please – I've got thrush!

It is possible that any woman, or man, suffering from repeated attacks of thrush is being reinfected by their sexual partner(s). That's why it's so important that sexually active sufferers get their partners treated too. Don't start having sex again until you have been given the 'all clear'. Women (or men) prone to thrush could try using condoms to minimize the chances of reinfection.

Help yourself to beat thrush

Self help works on the principle that you first restore the natural balance within your body, allowing your body to beat the overgrowth of candida and heal itself. You can help yourself to better health by adopting:

- an anti-candida diet
- an anti-candida lifestyle
- using natural remedies to treat and prevent further attacks.

Diet yourself better!

An anti-candida diet is one of the most important steps you can take to ridding yourself of thrush and, therefore, thrush-related cystitis (there's more about this in the next chapter and you'll find dietary details in some of the personal accounts in Chapter 16).

An anti-candida diet avoids food that contain yeast or moulds. That means giving up foods such as cheese, mushrooms and bread. Help yourself by eating lots of live yogurt. This contains *lactobacilli* organisms, which convert sugar into lactic acid. Lactobacilli are good for you because, once in the gut, they starve yeasts of the sugars they need to grow and they're great in the vagina for maintaining the slightly acidic environment that keeps thrush in check.

The anti-candida lifestyle

It's estimated that a third of the world's population now has candida and the problem is getting worse. The widespread use of antibiotics since the Second World War is partly responsible for this but, more recently, tights and synthetic fabrics, both of which prevent air from circulating around the crotch, have done little to promote vaginal health. Adopting an anti-candida lifestyle needn't mean denying yourself all of life's little pleasures, but it does mean that you may have to do certain things differently.

> I've had quite a bit of thrush since having a baby. I first noticed it a couple of months after the birth. I might have had it during my pregnancy as my baby got thrush in his mouth two weeks after he was born. Anyway I seem to get it a lot these days. It's itchy, makes my very sore and sometimes I get so swollen it's almost difficult to walk. I stopped using bubble baths because I was getting a lot of thrush. I mean you've only got to look at the colour of them to realize that they must be full of chemicals. They can't do you any good.

An anti-candida lifestyle is pretty much the same as an anti-cystitis lifestyle, which isn't surprising considering how closely the two conditions seem to be linked (Chapters 11 and 12 are packed with tips on how you can say goodbye to cystitis and thrush for good!).

Doing what comes naturally

Natural remedies, such as yogurt and lemon juice, tea tree oil and garlic, have all been very effective when used to treat thrush. Natural remedies are usually cheap, easy to use and have few or no side-effects. While they *may* not do any good, they cannot make the problem any worse, so all of them are worth a try.

Plain yogurt contains live cultures of lactobacilli. Naturally present in the body, lactobacilli organisms help to keep candida in check. Use it on a tampon or in a cap inside the vagina to soothe an existing attack or to ward off future infections. Lemon juice is acidic and again, used on a tampon or a cotton bud, may help restore the acid balance of the vagina. But tea tree oil and garlic are perhaps the two most effective thrush remedies, and they are described below.

TEA TREE OIL

My herbalist believes my cystitis to be caused by thrush so whenever I get an attack I just call her for some candida treatment. She's given me some antifungal pessaries and some tea tree oil drops to take internally. I know this will clear my cystitis up quickly.

Tea tree essential oil (from the plant *Melaleuca alternifolia*) is an extremely effective weapon in the war against thrush. It's often called a 'miracle oil' because it is non-toxic, non-irritant and a stronger germicide than carbolic. Tea tree oil, a pure and powerful plant extract, is both antiseptic and antifungal. Available reasonably cheaply from most good healthfood shops, it can be used in a number of different ways. Add a few drops to your bath water or use it directly on inflamed and itchy tissues. Because it is virtually non-irritant, even to the most sensitive tissues, you can use tea tree oil directly on your skin, but don't over do it. All essential oils should be used sparingly because they are so powerful. Put one drop of tea tree oil on a cotton bud, then use this to wipe it around the vagina and/or infected areas.

Tea tree oil pessaries and creams are available from larger healthfood shops or by post from the House of Mistry (see the Useful addresses section at the back of the book).

GARLIC

Like tea tree oil, garlic is extremely powerful against yeasts and fungi as well as bacteria. A recent report proved garlic to be more active against human ringworm (a fungal infection) than currently prescribed drug treatments. You can use it locally by inserting a peeled and pricked garlic clove into your vagina. Alternatively, eat as much raw garlic as you can to protect your body against candida.

Alternatives

Where conventional medicines have failed, it may be that natural or alternative therapies will succeed. There is a wide range of therapists practising alternative or complementary medicine. Alternative medicine has a high success rate with thrush because holistic practitioners usually treat the body as a whole rather than just the affected areas.

Alternative medicine may be very helpful in clearing up thrush-related cystitis and is definitely worth trying if you have had little success with standard cures. You can find out more about alternative therapies in Chapter 13.

6

Diet, diabetes and cystitis

Alcohol, food allergies and the anti-candida, anti-cystitis diet explained

I've found that my attacks are linked with diet. There seems to be a direct relationship between attacks and what I've eaten or drunk.

Centuries ago, before hospitals were commonplace and everyone had easy access to a GP, people often looked to their larders as a sort of food pharmacy. Of course, the therapeutic benefits of everyday foods are still there, it's just that fewer people know about them or rely on them in place of the laboratory-produced pharmaceutical drugs we have now. But many foodstuffs actually contain the same properties as the drugs we buy. Half a raw onion a day can boost your good HDL blood cholesterol by an average of 30 per cent. Only one anticholesterol drug (gemfibrozil) can do this, and then by an average of only 10 per cent!

Your diet can be a powerful weapon against illness. Similarly, eating foods that, unknown to you, disagree with you can make you unhealthy, unhappy, and prone to diseases. This chapter takes a look at the role certain foods play in preventing or causing cystitis.

What kinds of foods seem to cause the most cystitis?

Cystitis sufferers all over the world conclude that there are a few common foods that can trigger attacks of cystitis. If you haven't found out about these already through trial and error, you should make sure you know what they are so you can avoid them during a cystitis attack and, if possible, in the future too, to prevent recurrences.

Drinks that seem particularly bad are alcohol, tea and coffee, which are thought to irritate the lining of the bladder. These drinks are diuretics, which encourage the body to excrete more urine than normal. This can make you dehydrated, which is most undesirable during an attack of cystitis.

Remember, the first rule of cystitis management: *drink as much plain water as possible to help flush out the infecting bacteria.*

Becoming dehydrated only allows the infection to multiply more quickly in your concentrated urine.

If you get cystitis after drinking tea or coffee, try diluting them or avoid them altogether. Caffeine-free herbal teas are better for you, but can take some getting used to. Cammomile is a good one to start with – it's fairly mild-tasting and is known for its calming, healing properties.

Highly refined carbohydrate foods – typically white bread and white sugar – are also notoriously bad for cystitis sufferers and should be avoided, as should most processed foods. Not only are these kinds of foods of low value nutritionally, but they often contain chemical additivies that can bring on sensitivity (or allergic) cystitis. And they often contain added sugar, which encourages the growth of candida and can lead to cystitis (there's more about that at the end of this chapter in the anti-candida diet outlined there).

Avoiding the soft option

Little research has been done by the medical profession into what role diet plays in causing various illnesses. But one survey searching for a common factor among women suffering from recurrent urinary tract infections conducted at UCLA's School of Public Health pointed a finger at soft drinks, such as cola and lemonade. These increase urine pH, which might facilitate bacterial growth. They are of low nutritional value and either packed with sugar or artificial sweeteners, neither of which are good for your body. Avoid them where possible. Drink diluted natural fruit juices and water instead.

The trouble with alcohol

Alcohol and cystitis definitely don't mix! Not only does it irritate the bladder's delicate lining, alcohol also raises the urine's acidity and causes dehydration. And while a little alcohol in moderation can reduce the risk of heart disease, regular intakes raise the risk of colon and rectal cancer in both women and men. One study showed that larger drinkers in particular had greatly increased chances of developing cancer of the lower urinary tract and were more likely to develop this cancer the more lager they drank. Those who drank spirits were also at a higher risk for this cancer but, interestingly, those who drank wine were not. That's not to say that wine drinkers aren't at risk, however. A large-scale French study found that women who drank alcoholic beverages with meals were more likely to develop breast cancer than those who did not. The drinking of as few as three glasses of wine a week has been linked to a higher risk of breast cancer among women, notably those under the age of 50.

Some alcoholic drinks cause more of a reaction than others and so are worse for you than others. Red wine seems to be particularly bad for cystitis sufferers. If you can't give up alcohol completely, 'Long' drinks seem to be better for cystitis sufferers than 'short' drink lager or beer rather than whisky or gin. And to avoid dehydration have a soft drink – preferably plain or sparkling mineral water – before and afterwards.

> Drinking too much alcohol, or anything that will dehydrate me, can bring on an attack of cystitis. Sometimes on hot days in the summer when I haven't drunk enough I can feel cystitis coming on.
>
> My last attack of cystitis was caused by me getting very, very drunk the night before I left a job in Hong Kong. I went to bed without drinking any water and in the morning I had a 13-hour flight back to London. By the time I arrived, I was in such a state, I needed a really strong antibiotic to clear it up.

The cranberry juice cure

Cranberry juice is the perfect alternative soft drink for cystitis sufferers to sip. It has been known to relieve the symptoms of cystitis and other urinary infections for centuries. Indeed, references to cranberries in medical literature date back to 1860, although until a few years ago, doctors hadn't been sure just why these scarlet 'antibiotics' worked. Then scientists in Israel and Sweden discovered that cranberry and blueberry juice contain a compound that stops the bacteria that cause urinary infections from sticking to the walls of the bladder and other parts of the urinary tract. If these bacteria can't stick to healthy cells, they can't cause infections. And because the germs are unable to hang around in the bladder, they're simply flushed out of the body in urine, so they cannot multiply to dangerous levels and cause infection.

> I read somewhere that if suffering from cystitis, spicy foods and alcohol should be avoided and that drinking cranberry juice should be effective. If you just *have* to have alcohol, try vodka mixed with cranberry juice.

Almost all brands of cranberry juice available in the UK are heavily sweetened with sugar, so it's recommended that you make your own. To do this, just mix a little water with the juice of a few handfuls of fresh cranberries. Apparently the bacteria are even rendered helpless when the pure juice is diluted to one part juice per 100 parts water, so powerful is the agent!

American women swear by anti-cystitis cranberry juice capsules.

USA for many years and, thankfully, they can
tain. Made by both Solgar and Biocare, these
le from good healthfood shops, but if you have
em, you can get them by mail order from The
seful addresses section at the back of the book).

as other possible therapeutic benefits besides being a
against urinary tract infections. It can kill viruses and
kidney stones and deodorizes urine. And new research
confir ily half a cup of cranberry juice a day can ward off urinary
tract and bla der infections in women who are at high risk of infection.

Asparagus – not a luxury!

Did you know that asparagus is a good general tonic for all bladder and
kidney troubles? Herbalists advise sufferers to eat lots of it, as fresh as
possible. If you have a garden you could try growing your own. Eat the
succulent young tips or make a healing tea from the plant's fresh, raw
shoots. Add a handful of leaves to two cups of near-boiling water, then
allow to infuse overnight. Drinking two dessertspoonfuls morning and
night is supposed to relieve the symptoms of cystitis.

Food allergies

Allergy specialist Dr Jean Monroe claims that food seems to be the most
common cause of allergy-related cystitis. The foods that seem to be the
worst in this respect include those containing petrochemical additives (E
numbers) and sugary, yeasty foods that encourage candida.

Allergies can be permanent (or fixed), not disappearing with time, or
temporary (non-fixed), the body recovering with time. Milk allergy is
usually a short-term problem in that if it is avoided for a while the body
will sometimes tolerate it when it is reintroduced into the diet. Avoiding
the allergen (that which causes the allergic reaction) for a short period of
between one and six months is often enough to stop the symptoms of a
non-fixed allergy, provided your intake of these foods after this time is
low.

There are two reasons for so many people today being allergic to food.
It is likely that the human body functions best when fed a varied diet. We
should remember that our ancestors simply weren't used to eating the
same sort of foods week in, week out. Their diet depended on the
availability of certain foods in certain seasons. In short, their diets were
varied whereas today, because any kind of food can be shipped or flown in
from around the world, it's easy to eat the same foods all year round. And

many of these imported foods include highly allergenic food, such as citrus fruits, tea, coffee, cocoa and sugar. Also, since the Second World War, petrochemical additives (known as E numbers) have been added in larger and larger amounts to food. So, it's increasingly difficult to ensure that your diet is free from colourings, flavourings, preservatives, antioxidants, emulsifiers and stabilizers – all substances that can cause sensitivity reactions such as cystitis.

It can be hard to discover what you are allergic to because when you stop exposing yourself to the offending substance (say, a food or chemical) you may initially feel quite a bit worse. This is due to the 'hangover' effect created as the level of the allergen in your blood drops. It is only after five to seven days' abstinence, when the allergen has been completely removed from your body, that you will start to feel well. Also, when you re-expose yourself to an allergen, there may be a delay of up to 24 hours before symptoms reappear. In other words, you don't immediately get better as soon as the allergen is removed and you don't get worse immediately it is reintroduced. That's why many people don't know what causes their allergy; it's a catch-22 situation. Eating correctly, though, is very important in overcoming allergy problems; it helps the body begin to function optimally and deal with any other problems on its own, so it is worth doing the detective work.

How to find out what you're allergic to

Allergy specialists recommend eliminating certain foods from your diet one by one then gradually challenging your body by slowly reintroducing them. To ensure that the offending foods have been completely expelled from your body, you must cut them out for longer than the often-recommended five days – usually from a week to ten days. After eating allergens again, you should notice that your pulse quickens, although it may take up to 24 hours for the full effects to show up. By reintroducing certain foods one by one over a number of months, while carefully watching for the symptoms of your allergy to reappear, you should be able to pinpoint the real allergens.

If you think your cystitis could be allergy-related, you should consult your GP. Specialists do not recommend that anyone undertakes the elimination diet lightly. Go slowly, be careful and, if in doubt, consult an expert.

The anti-candida diet and cystitis

Food intolerance and food allergies are commonly associated with a candida problem. Candida causes food allergies when the invasive form of candida breaches the sieve-like lining of the intestines and allows larger molecules of food to pass into the blood. It's the presence of these larger molecules in the blood that leads to allergy problems. As the last chapter explained, candida or thrush is closely linked with cystitis. If you suspect that candida is behind your problem, it may be that you have a food allergy too. You can tackle both problems at once by following the anti-candida diet outlined below.

Foods to avoid

The basis of an anti-candida diet is avoiding yeast and sugar. But if you have cystitis too you will need to avoid acid foods as well. The no yeast, no sugar diet means avoiding fruit (which naturally contains a lot of sugar) while eating lots of vegetables and high-protein foods. Because high-protein foods are highly acidic they aren't the best sort of diet for the cystitis sufferer. The anti-cystitis diet, though, consists of mainly fruits and vegetables. You must cut down on your intake of animal protein and get this essential nutrient from its less acidic vegetable form – in pulses (peas, beans and lentils) and nuts. A dramatic change in your diet can take some getting used to, so take things slowly, one day at a time.

Remember, you won't have to stick to this diet forever. Once your symptoms improve, you can afford to slacken every now and then.

Start off first of all by cutting out added sugar from you diet. That means avoiding all the following sorts of foods:

- maple and golden syrup, malt and treacle and, as honey is a natural sugar, it is also on the forbidden list
- give up jam, biscuits, ice-cream (which is too cold for people with kidney/bladder difficulties anyway!), puddings, chocolate and other sweets
- don't drink sugary, fizzy drinks and fruit squash because, as we saw earlier, these can cause cystitis
- avoid dried fruits as they are very rich in natural sugars
- don't rely on artifical sweeteners to compensate – try to break your sweetness addiction completely
- cut out refined flour, which means white bread and anything made from white flour (pasta and pastry included!)

You are allowed small amounts of wholemeal bread and a few potatoes a week. And you may fill yourself up on unrefined carbohydrates, such as brown rice and vegetables! Also:

- wheat should be avoided as not only are wheat and wheat products highly allergenic foods but they are also highly acidic, like meat and dairy products (animal protein adds acid wastes to what your kidneys excrete and so can exacerbate infective cystitis).

My cystitis has been much better since I became vegetarian and stopped eating red meat. I gave up meat because I had what was called a spastic colon and I was quite constipated. I think this caused a lot of the bruising because I was so squashed up inside.

I have a really sweet tooth and I suspect that's why I get a lot of thrush. And nowadays whenever I get thrush I always get a sort of mild cystitis. Canesten pessaries and giving up sweets, white bread, Marmite and lager usually makes things OK again!

Foods to eat lots of

Eating too many acidic foods is harmful because it distorts the body's blood balance, making it overly acidic, causing arthritis and ulcers, for example. This in itself is unhealthy and can lead to many problems. Eating plenty of alkalinic fruits and vegetables can balance this. If you think this is too limiting, you'll be surprised how spoilt for choice you actually are! Salad vegetables such as lettuce, rocket, lamb's lettuce (or corn salad or mâche), watercress, radishes, raw carrots and celery can be piled high on delicious jacket potatoes. Or try turnips, beetroot and swedes with beans and peas, almonds and Brasil nuts, or fish and chicken to provide protein.

Leafy green vegetables, such as cabbage, Brussels sprouts, and broccoli, are good for you because they contain a high ratio of calcium to phosphorus. Try to buy organic vegetables wherever possible. Even though they are a bit more expensive, they are much better for you because food grown with fertilizers has an altered mineral content. And don't overcook, peel or shred fruits and vegetables or else they lose their vitamin content. For this reason, prepare salads and other raw foods close to the time when they are to be eaten to avoid losing out on valuable vitamins.

Yeast – the big problem

Many people are allergic to yeast and mould and their symptoms are greatly helped by a no sugar, no yeast diet. Candida sufferers should avoid yeast because it aggravates thrush (indeed, it is sometimes called a yeast infection).

Foods to avoid

The following can all encourage candida to multiply:

- all fermented drinks – this means alcohol
- all foods with a high mould content, for example, mushrooms and cheese or cheesy snacks (blue cheese, such as Roquefort, are the worst)
- foods with yeast in them, such as Marmite and yeast extract, and do not take brewers' yeast tablets or vitamin supplements that contain yeasts (if in doubt, check the label)
- food additives – monosodium glutamate, for example, is a yeast derivative and smoked meats and fish, sausages and hot dogs all contain additives, some of which are derived from yeasts, so beware
- all foods containing vinegar or fermented foodstuffs, which includes ketchup, mustard, soy sauce, pickles, relishes, salad cream and so on.

Garlic

Garlic is a powerful antibiotic and can attack the bacteria that can cause cystitis. So, eat as much raw garlic as you can! Crush it with oil and lemon juice and use it as a salad dressing or eat it blended with avocado, tomato, lemon juice and onions as a delicious dip.

Garlic can kill yeasts and fungi, too, so it's ideal for women who are prone to both cystitis and thrush.

My herbalist prescribed acidophilus and garlic tablets to replace the bugs in my gut wiped out by the courses of antibiotics. I have also used antifungal cream, which, together with the tablets, began to be effective this year. Recently I have also given in and abandoned tights and started to wear the dreaded suspender belt and stockings. Putting all this together has, I think, contained the problem, but I don't yet consider myself cured.

Fresh parsley, which is recommended in its own right as a good food for cystitis sufferers, will neutralize any odour of garlic on your breath. But if you really can't bear garlic, it's worth remembering that odourless garlic oil capsules are apparently just as effective as fresh garlic. Take four capsules, four times a day to fight and prevent infection.

Vitamins and minerals

Vitamins and minerals are vital for keeping diseases and ill-health at bay. Amazingly, adult women are almost *twice* as likely to suffer from allergies as men. Poor nutrition, causing low vitamin and mineral levels, makes allergies more likely, as do smoking, alcoholism and a poor general state of health.

Vital vitamins

If your diet is lacking in one or more essential vitamins, your body will suffer. For example, vitamin C is vital for building up your body's resistance to disease and also helps prevent allergies. Cabbages, tomatoes and citrus fruits are the richest sources of vitamin C, but it is found in all fresh fruits and vegetables.

Larrian Gillespie, an American urologist, advises women who have suffered from urinary tract infections to increase their intake of vitamin C. Vitamin C acidifies urine so that it is far more difficult for bacteria to thrive in it. As the body cannot store this vitamin and any excess is excreted in your urine, you will need to take plenty during an attack of cystitis as you are likely to be passing water frequently.

Drinking acidic drinks may help prevent occurrences of cystitis, although it's important to drink alkaline liquid (such as bicarbonate of soda) actually during an attack to reduce the burning pain. You may find it surprising to know that freshly squeezed citrus juices are only acidic until they enter the body, when they quickly become alkaline! Fruit is a most beneficial food for the kidneys because it contains components known to help sterilize the system. Eat plenty!

It's thought that people who have low levels of vitamin B_6, such as diabetics, are more susceptible to genito-urinary tract infections. Taking the Pill, a course of antibiotics and eating too much sugar all increase the body's need for vitamin B_6. As these are the main causes of thrush (candida) it looks like this vitamin is vital in preventing fungal infections too!

The vitamin B family, or vitamin B complex as it is known, has about 18 different members. Most of these are obtained from the same sources, so an inadequate diet will usually be deficient in *several* of the B vitamins rather than just one of them. Brewer's yeast, wheatgerm and meat are all rich in *all* of the B vitamins. Nuts, beans and lentils, and soya products are other good sources. Vitamin B_6 (pyridoxine) can be obtained naturally from most wholemeal products, oats, milk, fish and cabbage. Vitamin B_6 supplements are also available from all good healthfood shops. It is recommended that you take 100 mg of all major B vitamins daily to beat harmful bacteria.

Magic minerals

The minerals iron, magnesium and zinc have been pinpointed as being beneficial in preventing both thrush and cystitis. Among their numerous functions, they keep the blood and tissue fluids from becoming either too acidic or too alkaline. Zinc also helps to heal injured, irritated tissues. During a period, you lose about 30 mg of iron and so women are more likely to be deficient in iron than men. During pregnancy, the need for iron increases significantly. Green leafy vegetables, such as broccoli and spinach, are rich in iron, and the vitamin C that they also contain improves the absorption of iron from the intestine. That's two excellent reasons for including plenty of them in your diet!

Diabetes

Diabetes means that the body is unable to break down and use food in the usual way. This is because diabetics are either deficient in insulin (a hormone secreted by the pancreas) or because the body does not react properly to the insulin it produces. Insulin makes it possible for sugar (glucose) to enter the cells to be converted into energy. As this sugar can neither enter the cells nor be utilized as energy, it accumulates in the bloodstream. When the glucose level gets too high, sugar spills into the urine. The kidneys have to provide more urine to carry this level of glucose and the body needs to replace the excessive amounts of urine that the diabetic produces. Thus, severe thirst and an increased need to urinate are the earliest symptoms of the disease.

Diabetic women suffer from cystitis a lot. That's becaues the urine contains a lot of sugar, which encourages bacteria to grow. Diabetes may also affect the ability of the bladder to squeeze effectively, which is another reason diabetics are prone to cystitis. Because of the extra sugar in the vaginal walls, women with diabetes are also more likely to suffer from thrush which, in turn, can cause cystitis. Sugar in the urine, deposited on the vulva, provides food for the bacteria.

Undetected diabetes may be the source of a recurrent thrush and cystitis problem, so it's important to be tested for diabetes if this happens to you, especially if there is a history of the disease in your family. The presence of sugar in the urine can indicate diabetes, but your doctor should refer you to hospital for a full glucose tolerance test. Although diabetes is permanent, the illness can be treated. Some diabetics need daily injections of insulin, but in some cases, where the diabetic *is* capable of producing their own insulin, but only in small amounts, they will be able to control the problem by reducing their carbohydrate intake to a level that their own insulin supplies can deal with.

I began to suffer quite badly from cystitis when I was diagnosed diabetic nearly 30 years ago. I'd begun to feel unwell and lost a lot of weight, although at the time I couldn't understand what was wrong. I kept going to the doctor and eventually I underwent some tests which discovered I was diabetic.

I don't know why I became diabetic. The doctor did suggest that it might be because of a shock to my system. I had been running my own business and suffering from stress so he could be right. I started taking insulin tablets to try to control the diabetes, but these didn't work. After a year, I went onto insulin injections. I had to follow a strict diet, avoiding cakes, biscuits and all sweet foods.

It took a while for my body to adjust, but I definitely started feeling better, and putting weight on again. But I started getting cystitis a lot too. My doctor explained that diabetics are particularly prone to it. I must be getting proper infections because I always need antibiotics to clear it up – drinking gallons of water doesn't help. But over the last 18 months, I don't seem to have had it so often. This might be because I've been treated with a new antibiotic treatment called Unitor. Unitor is easy because you only have to take six tablets – one twice a day for three days. The symptoms usually clear up a day after taking the tablets. But, occasionally, it doesn't clear up and I have to go back for more.

As a diabetic I have to be careful about buying over-the-counter remedies. I can't take those cold relief powders, for example, so I doubt if I could have the cystitis remedies that the chemist sells.

The medical management of diabetes shows how closely diet and health are linked. The lesson to be learned from this is that looking carefully at your own intake of food could be the key to curing your cystitis.

7

Emergency!
How to cope when a
cystitis attack begins

The trouble with cystitis is that it usually catches you unawares. Knowing exactly what to do as soon as you feel the first twinge or two means you are half-way to beating cystitis.

Many sufferers are so familiar with the first signs of an attack that they are able to act immediately and so stand a better chance of curing themselves quickly. Following the emergency action plan outlined in this chapter will minimize the pain and discomfort of cystitis until you can get yourself to a doctor. It could even cure your cystitis as quickly as it starts.

When you feel the first signs of an attack

Start drinking! Drink at least 0.5 litre (1 pint) of plain water to help flush out any germs that are infecting your bladder and urethra. If you have cystitis you will feel like urinating even when you can't. This is why it's essential to keep drinking. If your kidneys are functioning normally, you'll soon be bursting to go and passing a full bladder is a lot less painful than passing just a few drips. If you force yourself to go, you could end up passing blood.

From now on, you must keep drinking as much water as you possibly can. Lemon barley water will help reduce the acidity of your urine. This means it won't burn the inflamed tissues of the bladder and urethra so you'll be in less pain. Avoid alcoholic drinks and coffee. Alcohol and the caffeine found in coffee are diuretics and encourage your body to excrete urine, which really won't help your condition at all. Tea also contains caffeine but very *weak* tea will gently stimulate you to pass water. And as long as you've been drinking lots of water and have plenty to pass, this may actually help you cope with cystitis.

Take two painkillers, such as aspirin or Ibuprofen, unless, of course, you're pregnant. Because these drugs are anti-inflammatories, they will help reduce the irritation in the bladder. The less inflammation there is, the less burning you will feel and the less pain. If you are pregnant and you suddenly develop cystitis, don't use *any* tablets without consulting your doctor.

Hotwater bottles can really help you cope with the pain. Fill them with really hot water and wrap them in a towel or T-shirt to stop the surface burning your skin. If you have two hotwater bottles, place one between your legs to numb the pain in your bladder and urethra. Prop the other hot water bottle on your back to soothe any kidney pains you might be feeling.

Get plenty of rest. Settle down on the sofa with your hotwater bottles and drinks lined up alongside you. Better still, go to bed. If an attack begins in the middle of the night you'll have hours to pass coping with your attack before the doctor's surgery opens, so keep yourself occupied. Take your mind off the problem by reading a good book. Alternatively, run a bath – relaxing in hot water will help relieve the pain.

> As soon as I get cystitis I put the kettle on. I keep filling it up and boiling water, for hot drinks and hotwater bottles. Waiting for the kettle to boil gives me something to do and takes my mind off the pain.

Twenty minutes later

Drink another 0.5 litre (1 pint) of liquid. Try to drink 300 ml (½ pint) of liquid or more if you can manage it every 20 minutes or so. 'Studies have been performed where bacteria were mechanically introduced into the bladders of volunteers,' says David Staskin, MD, an American urologist, 'Voiding just twice effectively sterilized the bladder.' Drinking and urinating flushes out the bacteria trying to build up in your bladder.

Stir a teaspoon of bicarbonate of soda into your second 0.5 litre (1 pint) of liquid. This will make your urine less acidic and ease the horrible burning sensation that goes with cystitis. (Note, however, that bicarbonate of soda should not be taken by people with heart conditions. Always check with your doctor first if you are in doubt.)

> I had a mild bout of cystitis at 60. One of my daughters told me to flush it out by drinking plenty of water mixed with a teaspoon of bicarbonate of soda. This worked like magic in a day. But it was a very mild attack, caught in the initial stages.

One hour later

Down another 300 ml (½ pint) of water mixed with a teaspoon of bicarbonate of soda. Follow this with 300 ml (½ pint) of plain water, herb tea or weak tea or lemon barley water.

Two hours later

Do the same again. Keep drinking, keep going to the toilet!

Three hours later

Drink another 300 ml ($\frac{1}{2}$ pint) of water mixed with a teaspoon of bicarbonate of soda. Again follow this with 300 ml ($\frac{1}{2}$ pint) of plain water, or weak tea or lemon barley water.

After about three hours, the initial pain of your attack should have subsided a little. As long as you keep drinking and going to the toilet, then you're coping! Repeat the painkillers as allowed (read the directions on the back of the packet carefully) and see your doctor. By this time, your cystitis may have improved so much that you might prefer to manage it yourself without a GP's help. If it hasn't and you're still in agony, make an emergency appointment with your doctors as soon as the surgery opens.

Be prepared for future attacks

I'm sure that keeping an anti-cystitis kit close by helps prevent me getting cystitis. I'm psychologically less likely to feel very grotty if I have some remedies to hand!

It's important to keep an emergency kit to hand to fight off any attacks in the future. The cystitis sufferer's motto really ought to be 'Be prepared!', especially as attacks often start up in the evening, hours before the doctor's surgery reopens.

Here's a checklist of your most essential items. Keep them all together somewhere where you can get to them without disturbing anyone else – you never know when you're going to need them:

- a tub of bicarbonate of soda
- hotwater bottle
- some painkillers, such as aspirin or Ibuprofen
- lavender essential oil – add a few drops to a hot bath
- an over-the-counter remedy, such as Cymalon, is a good idea, particularly if you've had success with it before as a cystitis cure
- a bottle of lemon barley water – drinking lots of it will dilute the urine, make it less acidic and soothe the urinary tract (you can make your own by boiling a cup of barley in 0.5 litre (1 pint) of water for 15 minutes, then pouring it through a sieve and flavouring the liquid with lemon juice)

- vitamin C tablets – taking about 1000 mg over 24 hours will acidify your urine enough to slow down any bacterial growth, so vitamin C therapy is an excellent idea if you can't get yourself to a doctor as quickly as you'd like to.

8

Cystitis and your doctor

As soon as you think you've got cystitis, you must get yourself to a doctor for a proper diagnosis and a cure.

Most women suffering from cystitis consult their family doctor or GP, making an emergency appointment. Don't let any doctor's receptionist convince you that you should wait any longer than a day for an appointment. If you do have an infection and it remains untreated, it could quickly rise to your kidneys and become very serious indeed, so insist that you be seen that day!

Any doctor you consult will want to make certain that you have cystitis rather than any one or more of the many other infections and complaints that cystitis can be confused with. So, once you've described your symptoms to your doctor they will almost certainly want you to supply a urine sample to be analysed at a laboratory by trained staff.

How to provide a midstream urine sample

Your doctor will ask you to provide a midstream urine sample (an MSU for short). This means that you begin to urinate to get a good flow going before you collect any of the urine in the sample bottle.

Supplying a midstream sample ensures that the urine you collect is bladder urine. Any bacteria present in the sample therefore strongly indicates a bladder infection. Micro-organisms that might have been lurking at the urethral opening or on nearby tissues will have been flushed away by the first bit of urine you passed. This is the theory, though few pathologists would claim this to be a foolproof test. You can help minimize the chances of getting a false positive by always washing your hands before giving a urine test.

Your doctor or the nurse will provide you with a sterile container to catch your urine sample in. But if you call the surgery from home and are asked to bring a sample with you, you must sterilize a jar yourself by putting it in a pan of boiling water for at least five minutes.

Testing time

Looking at a sample of your urine under a microscope the laboratory staff will confirm whether or not you are suffering from bacterial cystitis. If you are, then a 'significant' number of germs will normally, but not always, be found in that sample.

When a sample of urine is examined for evidence of infection, the staff will be looking for at least 100,000 micro organisms per millilitre of urine. Urine with less significant numbers of bacteria is said to be 'sterile', although, technically speaking, urine can never be completely sterile – there will always be some germs in your urine just as there will always be some germs on your hands, no matter how often you wash them.

As the usual request accompanying all urine samples is for 'microscopy, culture and sensitivity', the urine will also most likely by cultured as well as examined under a microscope. To do this, the sample is incubated overnight on a plate of nutrients to encourage any germs present to breed. Any bacterial colonies that spring up will then be inspected and detailed.

The sensitivity test done in addition to these two elements shows which antibiotics any germs found are sensitive to. This tells doctors which antibiotics are most likely to clear the infection.

The urine's acidity is usually tested as well. An acid urine with some pus but no bacterial growth indicates a mycobacterial infection, such as ureaplasma or mycoplasma. These are so commonly found in people's urine that a lot of laboratories see no point in testing for them. However, specialists in genito-urinary medicine believe that mycobacteria are significant in causing recurrent cystitis problems (for more about ureaplasma and mycoplasma, see Chapter 14).

How accurate are the tests?

As a rule, the type of urine test just described is the best way of accurately diagnosing 'true' or bacterial cystitis. It is particularly helpful in diagnosing urinary problems experienced by pregnant women, who may be unaware that they have an infection. Untreated urinary tract infections can cause problems in pregnancy and even lead to premature births. Any pregnant women attending regular antenatal check-ups can rest assured that her urine will always be tested for the first signs of infection, even if she hasn't noticed any obvious symptoms herself.

It is important to remember, however, that tests can give a *false* negative, which means that the numbers of the significant bacteria found in the sample you supplied amounted to fewer than the 100,000 micro-organisms per millilitre of urine required to label the test as positive. To maximize your chances of getting accurate results, make sure that you don't go to the toilet for at least two hours before the test. If you have cystitis you will undoubtedly find this difficult, but it will be worth it. And always ensure that you use a sterile container. Often, false *positives* are given when other bacteria come into contact with the sample, either from the jar itself or from your hands or body. If you've had acute cystitis before – that's a short, sharp, isolated attack that has responded well to antibiotics – you'll probably know how serious your cystitis is yourself. So, if you're worried that you have an *E. coli* cystitis infection and a test result indicates otherwise, ask your GP to repeat the test.

Any sample you give your doctor will have to be analysed properly at a local hospital laboratory, which can take up to a week. If your urine sample shows visible signs of infection – if it contains streaks or 'casts' of blood or pus or is very dark and/or smelly – your doctor really ought to prescribe a treatment (probably antibiotics) for you then and there. If they don't and you can't bear the thought of waiting for days before relief of your symptoms, simply ask your doctor to prescribe something straight away – they probably will.

What should normal urine look like?

I always know when I've got an infection. My urine is much darker and smellier. Normally my wee is a very pale yellow. It's clear and hardly smells at all.

Sometimes women panic when their urine looks a little different to usual. That's because one of the first signs of a urine infection is a change in the urine itself. Normal urine is not offensive and shouldn't be painful to pass. The urine you pass at the beginning of the day may be a little darker and more concentrated than that of the rest of the day, but typically, urine is pale yellow and clear rather than cloudy.

Some vitamin tablets, such as vitamin B, can make your urine darker than usual and make it smell much stronger than you may be used to, but otherwise, changes in your urine are usually a sign of illness and should be treated as such. If, for example, you become dehydrated as a result of diarrhoea, your urine will become darker and more concentrated. Brown or colourless urine may be a symptom of jaundice, which indicates that your liver or gallbladder isn't working properly. Pinky-red urine is a danger sign. It usually indicates an infection, although artificial food colourings, and sometimes natural ones such as beetroot, can occasionally discolour urine in this way. Don't take any chances – see your doctor right away.

Time for a change?

Some doctors are going to be very understanding and helpful when you've got cystitis, but sadly, some aren't.

My GP was so unhelpful the last time I got cystitis. I was in absolute agony but made it up to the surgery where I had to wait about an hour to be seen. I spent the whole time on the loo as it was impossible to do anything else. When I finally got to see my GP she asked me loads of questions and told me to stop fidgiting! I explained that I don't normally fidgit – I was trying to cope with cystitis! She said she couldn't give me any antibiotics until she'd taken a urine test. I dutifully supplied one. It was bright pink because, by this time, I was bleeding!

My GP took one look at the sample and said she would have to send it to our local hospital for analysis. 'Bloody urine', I thought! 'As if she needs any more proof than bright pink urine!' Anyway, to save time, I got a friend to drive me to the hospital to drop off the sample – I'd missed the surgery's morning collection. The hospital phoned through my results that afternoon and I finally got my antibiotics. But I don't think I'll be seeing that doctor again in a hurry!

If you find yourself making frequent visits to your GP about a cystitis problem and you're not happy with the treatment and advice you're being given, you can do something about it. Don't forget you can choose your doctor – you can change doctors if your present one doesn't take you seriously.

Other places you could go to for help

You don't have to rely on your doctor for help with cystitis. There are other clinics geared up towards treating this infection and they may be more sympathetic to your plight, particularly if you are a regular cystitis sufferer.

Well Woman clinics

Well Woman clinics encourage women to check and chat about their health. They were set up to help women with problems and medical conditions that GPs often don't have the time to advise on during normal surgeries. Well Woman centres help women who are in good health and who want to stay that way, so the doctors and nurses you see there will be able to counsel you on ways to prevent cystitis as well as ways to treat it.

Larger doctors surgeries run Well Woman clinics to treat a variety of women's problems, ranging from thrush and cystitis to tiredness and depression. They also offer help with problems connected with periods and the menopause. Ask at your hospital to find out whether or not there is one in your area. Your District Health Authority or Community Health Council will also be able to tell you where your nearest clinic is.

Genito-urinary medicine clinics

Genito-urinary medicine clinics, also known as special clinics, don't just treat people suffering from sexually transmitted diseases. They can also help women clear up common vaginal infections, such as thrush and gardnerella. Because they offer routine, on-the-spot testing, such clinics offer the best facilities for the accurate diagnosis of all genital infections.

These clinics are becoming increasingly busy, however, and many have limited resources. If they had to see all cases of cystitis they simply couldn't cope with the many other patients who need their specialist help. So, whether or not you will be welcomed at a genito-urinary clinic with a simple case of cystitis will probably be a matter of local policy. Some clinics only advise that people complaining of cystitis-like symptoms visit them if they have slept with anyone other than a regular partner in the last fortnight.

Genito-urinary clinics have lots of advantages. Many don't run an appointment system so you may be seen sooner there than at your doctor's surgery. As the results of your tests are given while you wait, if any infection is found you will be able to start treatment right away.

In Britain anyone can attend a special clinic without being referred by their own doctor – a situation that isn't echoed in some other countries. In the USA, Australia and New Zealand, for example, women with cystitis would not normally be accepted for treatment at special clinics. The address of your nearest clinic can be obtained from a family planning clinic, your local hospital or the *Yellow Pages*. It is best to telephone the clinic first to check whether or not they will be able to help you.

Genito-urinary clinics are very useful for detecting other genital infections. If you've been sleeping with a new partner and there's even a slight possibility that you might have contracted a sexually transmitted disease, head for one of these clinics straight away. Get your partner checked out, too. They might not have any symptoms, but may be carrying an infection that is causing your cystitis.

9

Treating cystitis

The most effective cure for a case of cystitis caused by *E. coli* or other enterobacteria is a course of antibiotics. Antibiotics can only be prescribed by a qualified doctor. That's why it's so important to visit a doctor at the first signs of cystitis, to ascertain the most likely cause of the attack and to receive the correct treatment.

Antibiotics

Antibiotics are the standard treatment for cystitis and other urinary tract infections. There are a great many antibiotics now on the market. If your urine has been cultured (see page 51), a sensitivity test will tell your doctor which antibiotics can effectively cure the bacteria causing the infection. Your doctor will need to know whether or not you are allergic to any antibiotics and, more importantly, whether or not you are pregnant. Antibiotics can harm an unborn child and most of them should be avoided in pregnancy.

Always complete the full course of antibiotics prescribed to you. If you don't, you greatly increase your chances of suffering a further attack. If all the bacteria aren't entirely eliminated from the bladder the *symptoms* of the infection may well disappear, but if an insufficient number of tablets are taken, the drug will not destroy *all* the germs infecting your bladder, just reduce them to a low level, so they will be quietly multiplying again for another attack. Several days later, therefore, you'll notice a recurrence of symptoms. This is not another attack, but the *same* infection that was never properly cleared from your system.

Not completing an entire course of antibiotics also causes your body to become resistant to their effects. Some women find it hard to take all the tablets prescribed; it's not that they deliberately stop taking the course, they just forget to take their tablets. That's why a one-dose treatment – simply taking one powerful dose of a drug as opposed to a full course – is an appealing option for most women. One-dose treatments are reported to work particularly well if you treat the cystitis at the earliest opportunity. An added advantage of one-dose treatments is that there's less chance of you getting thrush – itself often a cause of cystitis. If the infection fails to respond to a one-dose treatment, it might be that you have a more involved infection than simple cystitis and so you should consult your GP for more help.

Antibiotics for emergencies

Anyone with a long history of attacks should ask their doctor for a supply of antibiotics to keep for emergencies. These will be useful if an attack begins late in the evening or on holiday and will avoid any delay in obtaining a prescription. Medical experts agree that the sooner the antibiotic therapy commences the more effective it is likely to be.

Antibiotic treatment for sexual cystitis

My sympathetic GP allows me to stock up with antibiotics. If I take a double dose of tablets on the first tingling sensations of a cystitis attack, it disappears the same day.

Some women suffering from sexual cystitis have found that taking antibiotics after sex reduces the number of attacks they have. It's been proved that taking antibiotic and antimicrobial drugs after intercourse is a big benefit to women who suffer from sexually-related recurrent urinary tract infections. But women need not take these drugs continuously to keep the infections at bay – just taking them after sex is enough to ward off cystitis. This is good news for sufferers for whom sex spells urinary tract infection. However, the long-term use of antibiotics should only be a *last resort treatment*, one to call on when all other options have been explored. Sexually-related cystitis might simply be cured by changing some of your hygiene habits, both before and after sex. Doctors often fail to give women such simple self-help tips, even though such action is preferable to antibiotic therapy, as a first step.

It is also very important to avoid taking antibiotics on a long-term basis unless your doctor can confirm that you do *not* have interstitial cystitis. This is a type of cystitis that is actually caused by antibiotics. Long-term use of antibiotics can also cause thrush, which can aggravate the urethra and bring on cystitis-like symptoms. Also, taking low levels of antibiotics may encourage the development of antibiotic-resistant strains of infection! Read Chapters 11 and 12 for information on how you can avoid cystitis before turning to antibiotics.

The most commonly prescribed antibiotics

On the following pages are brief details of the antibiotics most commonly prescribed for cystitis. All of them have side-effects of one sort or another and you should be aware of them. And don't forget about candida (thrush). An overgrowth of this bacterium can arise as a result of taking antibiotics and it can be very difficult to rid the body of candida once it has taken a hold. To minimize the effects of antibiotics, ask your doctor to prescribe treatment for thrush to take concurrently. Thrush-susceptible cystitis sufferers may consider trying to 'drink themselves better' with plenty of water and bicarbonate of soda instead if they show no signs of significant numbers of bacteria in their urine.

Not all the drugs outlined below will be suitable for you. Their effectiveness often depends on how they react in your body. If you take several courses of them you could become resistant to them. Always ask your doctor's advice on exactly how they should be taken for maximum effectiveness. If you notice any side-effects, consult your doctor immediately. You may have to switch to another brand.

Bactrim and Septrin

These sulfa preparations contain a combination of trimethoprim and sulfamethoxazole – bacteriostatic drugs that stop micro-organisms from reproducing. They are particularly useful for treating urinary tract infections as the antibiotic effect accumulates and concentrates in the urine more than in body fluids or tissues.

The tablets carry an increased risk of kidney stones forming within the urinary tract, so counteract this tendency by drinking plain water. About three quarters of all reported side-effects are of skin reactions, such as rashes.

Amoxcyillin and ampicillin (penicillin)

Amoxycillin and ampicillin are penicillin derivatives effective against *E. coli* and *Proteus mirabilis* – although some strains of these cystitis-causing organisms are now resistant to them.

They are safe to take during pregnancy, but anyone allergic to penicillin should avoid both drugs. Even if you have not previously been allergic to penicillin, be careful as more people react to penicillin than to any other drug and allergies can develop at any time.

Furadantin and Macrodantin

These tablets contain an antiseptic called nitrofurantoin and may be used in low doses over a long period by people with chronic urinary infections. Taken with food or milk, they should not be prescribed during pregnancy.

Nitrofurantoin's side-effects include stomach upsets, nerve inflammation, jaundice or hepatitis-like symptoms, and possible liver damage.

Keflex

Keflex capsules should be taken at exactly the same time each day, with a large glass of water. Because this drug is more expensive, it is usually only prescribed when there is resistance to more commonly used drugs.

It can cause diarrhoea, heartburn, rashes and dizziness. Take care if you are very sensitive to penicillin as you may also react to Keflex.

Tetracycline

Due to the widespread use of this drug, a growing number of strains are resistant to it. So, if another effective antibacterial drug can be used in its place, you may consider avoiding tetracycline.

Tetracycline should be taken on an empty stomach when it can be best absorbed into the urine. It should never be taken with milk or other foods high in calcium as this negates the drug's effect.

Children, pregnant women and breastfeeding mothers shouldn't take tetracycline. The drug may cause skin reactions, such as rashes, which may persist for weeks or months after the course has been completed.

Erythrocin

Erythrocin contains the antibiotic erythromycin, which is safe to take during pregnancy, although it should not be taken by children.

The drug can cause stomach upsets and allergies and should not be taken by anyone suffering from liver disease.

Alternatives to antibiotics

Antibiotics aren't the only cure for a cystitis attack. There are lots of successful alternative treatments (see Chapter 13). There are also medicines that your doctor can prescribe as an alternative to antibiotics. They have an antiseptic action on the urinary tract and are effective against *E. coli* bacteria.

Pyridium is one such treatment. Containing phenasopyridine hydrachloride, it should be taken until the infection has cleared. Taking Mictral granules (nalidixic acid with sodium citrate and bicarbonate) dissolved in water, three times a day for three days has been proved as effective in treating cystitis as a longer course of antibiotics, such as co-trimoxazole (Septrin).

Remember, however, that like all powerful drugs, these treatments can have side-effects. Pyridium can turn your urine orange or red, which may stain your clothing, and can also cause a dry mouth, drowsiness or dizziness. Mictral can cause stomach problems, disturbed vision, anaemia and blood changes. And neither preparation should be taken during pregnancy.

Over-the-counter remedies

There are several preparations that can be bought at your local chemists to alleviate the symptoms of cystitis and sometimes cure them.

The good thing about remedies such as Cymalon and Cystemme is that they relieve the terrible burning pain associated with cystitis. They work in the same way as bicarbonate of soda, neutralizing the urine's acidity. Sometimes this is all the help a sufferer needs until the inflammation subsides of its own accord.

These over-the-counter remedies claim to relieve cystitis in 48 hours, so if you are still in pain after this time, see your GP immediately. They can be useful to have to use in emergencies and they can help to ease the symptoms of cystitis until you can get a doctor's appointment. They can't affect bacteria, so you won't affect the results of your urine test by taking them.

I've never seen the doctor about my cystitis because it's never been that bad. Anyway, I don't like to take antibiotics if I can help it. I've never bled, it just feels like I need to go to the loo when I've no urine to pass, so it's more unpleasant than painful. I usually drink loads and loads of water until it goes away. I buy one of those over-the-counter remedies from the chemist and I usually feel fine after a couple of days.

Bicarbonate of soda and mist. pot. cit.

Lots of women say they rely on good old-fashioned bicarbonate of soda to cure their cystitis. This is an alkaline powder that can be bought for not very much in supermarkets and chemists.

Drinking half a pint of water mixed with a teaspoon of bicarbonate of soda will make your urine less acidic. This helps to relieve the pain of cystitis because alkaline urine reduces the burning sensations felt in an inflamed bladder and urethra.

An attack always starts like this. I wake up in the morning and feel an urgency to go to the loo. I'm so familiar with the symptoms now I find myself thinking 'Here we go again'. When I pass urine it stings and my bladder goes into spasm. I get this shooting pain inside and feel like I need to go again. I don't because I know it will only hurt even more. I start drinking ... weak orange juice mixed with a teaspoon of bicarbonate of soda, on the hour every hour. The pain usually goes by lunchtime.

Mist. pot. cit. (potassium citrate) is another over-the-counter remedy that chemists make up for cystitis sufferers. Some women find it helps relieve their symptoms and can cure an attack. Almost everyone agrees, though, that it tastes quite disgusting! Try it – if you can stomach it – because it may well work.

I always use potassium citrate with hyacinth which any chemist will make up for you. I suffered badly with recurrent cystitis for quite some time. None of the over-the-counter packets (Cystemme, Cymalon, etc.) ever seemed to work. But potassium citrate does. You simply drink it in a glass of water whenever you feel the first twinge!

The first time I got cystitis I bought an over-the-counter remedy called Cymalon. But it took about five days to clear up. I drank gallons of water too, so that might have helped. The next time I got it I went into an alternative health-type of chemist and asked them for something for cystitis. They gave me potassium citrate they'd made up themselves. It made me feel quite sick to take it but it cured it in a day or two. I didn't have to see my doctor.

It's your choice

Remember, you *do* have a choice about which remedies you take. You will feel much better psychologically by only taking those you feel comfortable with. There are numerous alternatives to conventional treatments, such as acupuncture and acupressure, psychic healing and reflexology (see Chapter 13 for more). And, one last word of advice: don't take any over-the-counter remedies if you are, or think you might be, pregnant. See your doctor instead.

10
Specialist help

Repeated attacks of cystitis need further investigation than a simple urine test. If you suffer from recurrent cystitis, your doctor can arrange for you to have special tests to help get to the root of the problem. About one in ten of all women who visit their doctor with cystitis are referred to hospital for specialist assessment and investigations. Referred cases are seen by a urologist, the medical term for an expert in the urinary system.

What a urologist will do

A urologist can't begin to treat you until they have built up a detailed picture of your particular problem. So, on your first visit, you will be asked lots of questions about yourself.

It's important to give the urologist as much information as you can. They need to know about your periods, your diet and your sexual history. Gynaecological disorders, such as vaginitis and/or thrush, need to be ruled out as contributing factors. The urologist will want to know about your health in general to ensure that you do not have a more serious problem, such as tuberculosis of the bladder or cancer of the bladder. Neurological diseases, such as multiple sclerosis, sometimes present with lower urinary tract symptoms, including frequency and urgency, so these, too, need to be ruled out.

A urologist will also want to know how long you've been affected by cystitis, your symptoms, what tends to trigger an attack and what, if anything, makes it better. Once they've conducted this investigation, they will probably do a microscopy, culture and sensitivity test on your urine, particularly if you have recently had an acute attack.

Other tests

If you suffer from repeated attacks of cystitis, your specialist will want to rule out the possibility that you have any anatomical abnormality of the urinary tract. They will want to check whether or not your urethra is constricted and that there is no blockage, such as those caused by chalky deposits, which can build up inside the kidneys or bladder (a bit like fur in a kettle), known as stones. Above all they will want to find out whether or not your urinary system is working properly and the best way to do this is by means of an intravenous pyelography or urethography.

Intravenous pyelography

An intravenous pyelography provides doctors with a series of X-ray pictures of the urinary tract.

You mustn't drink any liquids for several hours before the pyelogram is done. Then, liquid containing chemicals that show up on X-rays is injected into the bloodstream. It travels around the body until it is absorbed by the kidneys (this may take several hours). X-ray pictures are taken as the chemical works its way through the kidneys, down the ureters and into the bladder.

The X-ray pictures taken will show up any kidney stones (large urinary stones may need removing; smaller ones may find their own way out) and any defects, such as *ureteric reflux* (that's when urine flows backwards from the bladder back into the ureters) and *reflux nephropathy* (when urine flows backwards from the ureters into the kidneys).

A cytoscopy

If your urinary tract appears to be functioning normally, your specialist may decide to look more closely at your bladder, to see if there is any abnormality there. One procedure used to do this is called a cytoscopy and it is usually done under general anaesthetic.

An instrument called a cytoscope (which is a bit like a periscope) is inserted into the urethra and through to the bladder. A special eyepiece allows doctors to look for signs of inflammation and other problems.

A cystoscopy will pick up anatomical defects, such as a cystocele obstructing the bladder. A cystocele is the term used for when the bladder has prolapsed into the vagina – a cause of cystitis. Pressure on the bladder prevents it from being completely emptied, so any remaining urine in the bladder stagnates and can become infected.

Micturating cystogram

This is a series of X-rays taken while the bladder contracts and empties. The pictures clearly show the action of the bladder during urination. A micturating cystogram is often done following an intravenous pyelography when chemicals visible on X-ray are already in the bladder. However, sometimes the chemical solution is passed directly into the bladder through a fine tube inserted into the urethra, specifically to observe the bladder rather than the rest of the urinary system.

Bladder function tests

These tests are a bit like a bladder MOT. They help doctors to get a clearer picture of how well your bladder is working. They have three parts:

1 *Testing bladder volume* You are asked to urinate into a bowl, then a catheter is inserted through the urethra into the bladder to draw off any remaining urine and the total volume of urine is measured.
2 *Testing pressure* Pressure-measuring devices are attached to the catheter to measure the strength of the empty bladder's muscular contractions.
3 *Testing pressure during urination* When you have a full bladder, a catheter containing pressure-measuring devices is inserted into the urethra to measure the pressure exerted by the bladder as you pass urine.

What happens next?

Not all the tests described here will be done in every case. They may also be done in different orders. Sometimes these tests will need to be repeated to monitor progress or to pick up any complications.

The tests described immediately above check whether the bladder is emptying itself fully. They also test bladder tone and check how efficiently the bladder muscles are working. Poor bladder function can be improved by exercise and a good diet, so if corrective surgery on the bladder is suggested, do not agree to this without first finding out what side-effects such surgery might have. If necessary, ask for a second opinion. There is always the chance that bladder surgery could make any existing problem worse.

The surgical option

Urologists often try to correct urinary tract abnormalities with surgery. Experts seem to be divided as to how effective surgery is. Unconfirmed reports have claimed success for treatments such as *urethral dilation* and *internal urethrotomy* (making a slit in the urethra to help it drain). But other urologists believe that these operations have a very doubtful place in the treatment of women with recurrent symptoms.

Urethral dilation
Urethral dilation widens the urethra and is a fairly common procedure offered to women suffering from repeated attacks of cystitis. The logic behind the operation is that the cystitis-like symptoms occur because the urethra is too narrow. Thus, urethral dilation is also offered to women whose urethras have become constricted or narrowed by scar tissue that has built up as a result of repeated attacks of cystitis. In such cases, often only the constricted section of the urethra is widened. Whatever the reason

for the operation, urethral dilation is always done under general anaesthetic. It can be painful and may not always work. Some women have even been advised to have it done every six months! Here are two women's accounts of how this operation affected them.

I'd spent about three years suffering from cystitis, the treatment for which kept causing other problems such as gardnerella or thrush to flare up. Then one doctor examined me and said, 'I can feel a kink in your urethra. That's where the problem is!' I felt such relief just knowing what it might be and that something might be done about it.

He managed to get me on a hospital short list and I had a urethra dilation. The results were incredible! I suddenly felt like I could get a good flow going when I urinated whereas I don't remember being able to do this before. Having had so much cystitis, I had felt scarred and permanently uncomfortable. But after the operation it was almost as if I could feel germs flushing out of me. I wasn't cured completely but whenever I got cystitis again, I could cure it myself rather than resort to antibiotics. If I felt the first twinges of cystitis coming on I would be able to flush the attack away by drinking lots of water and bicarbonate of soda whereas before the operation any cystitis would go straight to my kidneys.

When I married and started having sex regularly, cystitis became a recurrent problem. I seemed to be getting an attack every few months. Eventually I saw a specialist and had an operation to stretch my urethra. This helped initially, but after a while I began to suffer again.

Larrian Gillespie, an American urologist, disagrees with the practice of urethral dilation. She believes that this treatment cannot possibly work and she is also against the current method used to measure the width of the urethra. She believes that the sphincter muscles will automatically contract around any catheter or probe placed into the urethra, that is, that this simple, involuntary muscle reaction gives false information about the size of the urethra. Dr Gillespie believes that rather than curing cystitis, dilation can actually, on the contrary, harm recurrent sufferers. The procedure, she believes, can cause tiny tears in the urethra that then scar, possibly eventually causing constriction – the opposite effect to that intended. However, many women who have undergone this treatment to rid themselves of recurrent cystitis *do* report that it has worked.

I'd been suffering attacks of cystitis since I began having a regular sexual relationship with my boyfriend. Looking back on it now, all the attacks I've ever had have been linked with sex, but at that time I didn't recognize the link. I was living in Germany and my doctors did a series of tests to try to find the cause of the problem.

I'm still traumatized by the cytoscopy I had. Apparently if I'd had it done anywhere else I'd have had an anaesthetic, but in Germany I wasn't offered any pain relief at all.

The urologist stuck a tube up inside my urethra and put a cytoscope inside. He had a good look round, then pumped my bladder with water and made me sit in the waiting room for ten minutes. I was bursting to go to the loo and in agony. Then I had to go to the loo while they measured how quickly the urine flowed out. I bled for days afterwards!

As a result of this test, the urologist said that my urethra was obstructed by a small lump. The urine stagnating behind it was causing infections to develop. The lump was removed under general anaesthetic and my urethra was widened. I noticed that after the operation my urine flowed out faster; it didn't take me so long to go the loo. Yet because I'd had to have a catheter after the operation, I immediately got cystitis. I had to take antibiotics to clear it up.

I feel quite strongly that the operation did not help but that it made matters worse. In fact, I'm convinced that it damaged me in some way. Now I find that even if there is no infection, unless I drink large quantities of liquid every day, urinating is painful.

So, although cystitis sufferers can find that urethral dilation does help them, particularly where there is an anatomical problem involving the urethra or bladder, you are advised to think carefully before booking yourself in for the operation. This goes for the other surgical treatments you may be offered, including one to stretch the urethral opening. In some women, this opening may be situated in or unusually close to the entrance to the vagina, so they are particularly susceptible to cystitis after intercourse.

Think of surgery as your last resort and remember that prevention is better than cure. There are many essential self-help tips in the next two chapters; don't even think about going for an operation until you have tried every one of them!

11

Self help: helping yourself
to a happy ever after

I don't think there's any one remedy for cystitis, but a range of options. Sufferers have to find out what suits them. I don't attribute my 'cure' to one remedy alone. I've changed my diet and my clothing – I no longer wear tights and tight trousers. And I also use special herbal remedies. These three things have helped to keep my cystitis at bay.

This chapter is not about trying to cure yourself of a fully blown attack. It's about preventing recurrent attacks once your cystitis is being treated. As many women already know, the only way to keep cystitis at bay is to help yourself. And the great thing about helping yourself to a happy ever after is that you become in control of your own health.

But what are the most crucial prevention tips for helping to keep cystitis away? Your four-point cystitis-avoidance programme is to:

- drink plenty of fluids so your body makes plenty of urine
- make sure you obey the call of nature as soon as you need to and empty your bladder completely each and every time you go to the toilet.
- keep germs away from the urethra
- take care to avoid becoming sore and bruised during sex.

Because cystitis is often so closely linked with sex, a complete sexual cystitis-avoidance programme is detailed in the next chapter. It will be of great help to those women for whom intercourse invariably triggers off an attack. But don't rush straight to Chapter 12 without reading the self-help tips in this chapter. The points made here are important for *all* cystitis sufferers.

A proven success

Medical research has tried to come up with foolproof self-help tips for cystitis sufferers. And scientists have proved that helping yourself can be a big success. One study in America (Adatto, et al.) looked at how the following cystitis-avoidance programme worked for 84 cystitis sufferers. The women were advised to:

- urinate every two hours, and always within ten minutes of sex
- drink at least 1.7 to 2.5 litres (3 or 4 pints) of liquid every day
- use plenty of lubrication during sex
- wipe from front to back after going to the toilet.

The group kept to this cystitis-avoidance programme for a whole year. Only 15 per cent of the group experienced a reinfection within six months, a much lower incidence than normally would have been expected. These steps are therefore pretty essential in helping to prevent urinary infections taking hold again.

Important

If you are drinking more, you must also go to the toilet more to prevent your bladder overstretching. And drinking *huge* amounts of liquid may strain your kidneys, so don't overdo it!

Good toilet habits

Learning good toilet habits can make all the difference for women prone to bladder problems. Often these have to be relearned. Chapter 4 described how many recurrent cystitis sufferers confessed that they habitually put off going to the toilet. Never, ever defer urination. Go to the toilet *whenever* you feel the need – hanging on can encourage an attack of cystitis. Urine stagnating in the bladder becomes a breeding ground for harmful bacteria. Obeying the call of nature as soon as it is felt will stop this happening.

It's also important to empty your bladder *completely* whenever you go. If you find this difficult, try counting to 20 when you *think* you've finished, then try again to push out the last few drops. This practice has been proved to help cystitis sufferers keep free from infection.

Wipe the right way

Each and every time you go to the toilet, wipe yourself from front to back. This way you'll be wiping germs *away* from your urethra. Never wipe yourself from back to front. If you do, you'll be wiping bacteria towards and possibly into the urethra.

Using plain, preferably unbleached toilet paper can make a difference too. Coloured toilet tissue contains chemical dyes that may irritate your urethra. Forget moist (chemically impregnated) toilet tissue for the same reasons. When the highly sensitive mucous membranes around a woman's vulva come into contact with irritant chemicals, they can easily become inflamed. This could trigger an attack of vaginitis or cystitis – or both.

Chemicals can cause cystitis

Doctors specializing in allergy and environmental medicine are seeing an increasing number of women complaining of vaginitis and urethritis caused by 'feminine hygiene' products, such as vaginal deodorants, deodorized sanitary towels and tampons. The surest way to avoid an allergic reaction to such products is simply not to use them.

Our bodies aren't meant to be squeaky clean. No amount of disinfectant will remove the germs that live and breed on the human skin. Be hygienic, but only use water around your genitals. Your vagina is a self-cleaning organ – it doesn't need douching or deodorizing. Douching is particularly harmful as it can actually introduce infectious bacteria, such as *E. coli*, into the vagina.

A smelly vaginal discharge indicates that an infection is present and this needs treatment – it shouldn't be masked with vaginal deodorants. These products contain a chemical cocktail of perfumes and disinfectants that can irritate the delicate vaginal membranes and possibly even trigger an infection. Vaginal deodorants are a totally unnecessary and potentially harmful product.

The thing to remember, therefore, is be clean, but don't be obsessed. Keep the genital area clean by washing with plain water morning and night. (Overwashing is a problem in itself as this may disturb the natural biological defences of the vagina.) Wash the anus with a little pure unperfumed soap, then rinse with plain water. There's no need to use soap around your vagina or urethra – plain water is enough. Soap is alkaline and can upset the delicate acid alkaline balance of the mucous membranes of the vagina, which in turn can lead to other problems, such as thrush.

Banish bubbles from the bathroom

It's not just soap that can irritate your nether regions. Using bubble baths or oils in your bath puts your vagina, urethra and bladder at risk. Even shampoo suds from washing your hair in the bath can be bad for you, especially if you already have a cystitis/urethritis problem. Recent American research linked the rise in the number of people suffering from cystitis-like symptoms to the increasing use of chemically loaded bath additives. Never add anything to your bath that you wouldn't put in your mouth. If you stick to this rule you shouldn't run into any problems.

Take showers instead of baths whenever possible. If you don't have a shower, sitting in your bath pouring jugfuls of warm water over your body will keep you as clean as any long hot soak in the tub, and is kinder to your vagina.

Healthy clothing

It's true: what you wear can seriously affect your health! It's long been known that wearing tights and nylon pants encourages vaginal thrush. In fact since women started wearing nylon tights, the incidence of thrush has soared. If getting thrush gives you cystitis, read on.

Nylon tights (and pants) retain the body's heat. Unlike cotton, nylon fibres won't let air pass through. And because nylon doesn't absorb moisture, tights and nylon pants, and even very tight trousers, can make your crotch warm and wet – just the sort of environment that thrush likes best.

E. coli, which causes cystitis, also thrives in warm, moist conditions. Don't make your vagina a breeding ground for bacteria. You can avoid getting thrush and cystitis by wearing:

- cotton underwear
- stockings, not tights, or open crotch tights (good hosiery shops sell these)
- skirts instead of trousers whenever possible.

Loose-fitting linen, cotton or wool trousers let air circulate around the vagina. Cold fresh air destroys fungus spores and bacteria, so wearing no pants at all is a good idea, especially when you are recovering from cystitis or a vaginal infection.

Taking care about what you wear may only be necessary for a short while. Once you break a recurrent cystitis pattern you may find you're able to wear whatever you like with no further problems.

Checklist of cystitis-avoidance tips

- *Always wear cotton underwear* Nylon pants and tights don't absorb moisture. Yeast and bacteria like *E. coli* thrive in a warm, moist environment, causing problems such as thrush and cystitis.
- *Never use perfumed soaps or bubble bath* Don't add anything to your bath other than salt, bicarbonate of soda or pure essential oils. Chemical bubble baths and so on can irritate and inflame the urethra, causing cystitis.
- *Always wipe from front to back with dry toilet paper* Preferably, use unbleached and definitely not coloured toilet paper.
- *Don't use other people's towels or flannels* Germs can spread this way.

- *Use towels instead of tampons* Tampons can actually cause cystitis. One survey analysing lifestyles of cystitis sufferers found a definite link between cystitis and tampons.
- *Never ignore the desire to go to the toilet* This can actually cause cystitis, so make sure you go whenever you feel the need.
- *Empty your bladder completely every time you go to the toilet* You'll help to prevent a residue remaining in the bladder that will encourage infection to develop.
- *Practise pelvic floor muscle exercises – regularly!* These improve pelvic muscle tone and the blood supply to your pelvic area, which helps heal damaged tissues.
- *Always drink plenty of fluids* This will help to keep flushing the bladder free of germs so bacteria won't be able to build up.
- *Always empty your bladder after sex* For lots of women, this single tip keeps them cystitis-free. (There are more tips on how to avoid sexually-related cystitis in the next chapter.)

> Whilst all of the cystitis attacks I have ever had have been after sex, I think that there are other factors as to whether cystitis follows. I am sure that moving to a warmer flat has helped reduce the number of attacks I was getting. Also, I'm scrupulous about personal hygiene these days. I drink a large glass of mineral water or a cup of green tea before going to bed (if sex is on the cards). After sex, I get up immediately and go to the toilet. I then wipe over the urethra entrance with toilet paper, moistened with warm water. I find this soothes it. The next day, I make sure I drink as much as possible. This is all very troublesome, but it is worth it as I seem to have conquered it.

12

Cystitis-free sex

It got to the stage when I'd begun to associate sex with doctors' surgeries. You stop wanting sex if it means antibiotics and doctors' waiting rooms all the time.

Sex became a scientific experiment. I'd have sex and wouldn't know whether the next morning I was going to wake up with itching, distress, soreness, pain or whether it was going to be another visit to the special clinic. If, during penetration, my partner's penis hit an area of soreness, I would immediately clamp up. I would only have to be rubbed or touched in a certain spot and I would just know that I was going to get cystitis. So I'd end up anticipating it and that caused so much fear I really went off sex for a while.

Sadly, very many women have come to associate sex with cystitis. Having sex should be a pleasure, but when you get cystitis, sex becomes a pain. And the only way to beat the pain is to break the link between cystitis and sex. Ignore any doctor who tells you that the cure for cystitis is to give up sex altogether. This is not practical and is very bad advice. It is possible to have cystitis-free sex. Read on to find out how.

Good clean fun!

The best way to avoid sexual cystitis is to wash yourself regularly. That means at least once a day. It's particularly important to wash before and after you have sex. If you suffer a lot from urinary tract infections, this isn't just a suggestion, it's an order!

Bacteria can easily be transferred from person to person during sex and then pushed into your urethra. And germs can hang around your bottom after a bowel movement so beware.

I know that cleanliness is really important in avoiding cystitis. I think because women have periods they're used to cleaning their bodies and being hygienic. I don't think men bother much about washing. I mean, just think what some men put in your vagina. If you look at their nails and think where they've had their hands before, it's not surprising they can give you cystitis!

71

Ask your lover to wash too – and it's not just a matter of keeping your genitals clean; germs are more likely to be introduced into the urethra by dirty hands during foreplay. Uncircumsized men should take extra care and wash under their foreskins, as bacteria like to lurk in warm, dark places.

Sometimes women are embarrassed to wash before sex simply because to stop so abruptly might kill the spontaneity of a moment of passion. Leaving your lover's side to wash straight afterwards can seem cold and clinical too. But there really is no bigger passion killer than cystitis. It's better to stop and wash than to go ahead and go down the old cystitis route yet again!

Washing the water bottle way

Often it's not practical to wash before sex every time without a shower attachment to hand or a bath at close quarters. Cystitis sufferers should keep a clean plastic water bottle by their toilet – the type you can buy mineral water in will do. Sterilize the bottle by rinsing it with a mild solution of the fluid used for sterilizing baby's bottles, then fill it with cold, boiled water. Then all you have to do is pour the water over the whole genital area before sex as you sit on the toilet. Easy! Make sure that water runs from the vagina down to the anus – avoid flushing bacteria towards the urethra.

Not only does washing with cold water after sex (using the bottle method again) reduce the likelihood of getting bacterial cystitis; it also reduces the likelihood of getting non-bacterial cystitis, the type that arises when the tissues of the vagina and urethra become inflamed and sore. That's because cold water reduces swelling and bruising in the area and lets the tissues heal themselves more quickly.

> I read about the bottle method of washing several years ago. It was invaluable when I was a student. I lived in a house where the loo and the bath were in separate rooms. Keeping a full bottle of cold water by the loo kept me cystitis-free for years. Now I have my own place and I can wash myself with the shower attachment, either sitting on the loo or crouching in the bath. But if I'm caught away from home and I need to wash, I just dampen a wad of toilet paper under the tap and wipe myself that way. I figure this method of keeping clean is better than nothing.

Bidets are not a good idea as sitting in a shallow puddle of water is potentially hazardous. Germs can easily float from the anus into the vagina and urethra. Bidets have several good uses, but washing your bottom is not one of them.

Sexual positions

Some sexual positions may put pressure on the bladder and so cause inflammation. And certain sexual positions are better than others for avoiding pressing on and rubbing the bladder. But a position that works well for one woman with one partner may make her sore with another partner – there aren't any hard and fast rules. Experiment a bit and have fun!

You may experience a cystitis attack when you change sexual partners. This might be because your system is accustomed to the bacteria of one sexual partner and your body may have trouble adjusting to the bacteria of another person. Very often it's not just a case of adjusting to a new partner's different ways of doing things, but of getting used to how your bodies react to each other and generally fit together.

When you start a sexual relationship with a new partner, it's likely that you'll be having sex more frequently. A new lover might be less aware of positions that make you sore and you, in turn, may feel less inclined to spell out your sexual preferences. Don't be passive or hesitant about telling your partner about your needs. Make sure your partner knows which sexual positions you prefer to keep you cystitis-free and happy.

Honeymoon cystitis

I have suffered from cystitis a few times in the past. The first time ever on honeymoon – on the first night! I didn't know what it was at the time.

Years ago, sexual cystitis used to be called honeymoon cystitis, because traditionally, it was on her honeymoon that a woman experienced a burst of vigorous sexual activity! Many women were virgins on their wedding nights. Nowadays, many women have sex – and cystitis – years before their honeymoon's booked!

But why should a period of sexual activity trigger an attack? And what is it that makes some women more susceptible to sexual cystitis than others? A recent survey compared the sexual habits of a group of cystitis sufferers with non-suffering women to try to find out just what sort of sex most typically brings on cystitis. It discovered that some women from each group reported burning, irritation or soreness after sex, even if they had sex regularly. But there did seem to be a link between infrequent sex and irritation after sex – that is, the women who had sex irregularly suffered from more soreness (and thus more cystitis/urethritis) than those who had sex more frequently.

When I haven't had sex for a while, I sort of turn off it. I find it's harder to get aroused and I often end up sore. But the more I have sex, the more I want to have sex. Having sex every day, on the other hand, is much easier. It makes me feel turned on and I never feel bruised. It's as though your body toughens up to the continuous activity!

The wetter the better!

If you haven't had sex for a while, it makes sense to take it slowly and use a lubricant, like KY Jelly. This is a water-soluble lubricant that you can buy over the counter at any chemist. Almond oil works just as well, if not better. It's ideal for sensitive skins as it's a totally natural substance. You can also buy this from chemists (a small bottle is inexpensive and lasts a long time – a little oil goes a long way!).

Using a lubricant during sex helps to prevent soreness and bruising. The urethra can get bruised during sex because it is so near the vagina. When it gets bruised, tiny cracks may appear in the walls of the urethra or scars from previous cystitis attacks may reopen, making urinating painful. Make sure you are sexually aroused before you have intercourse. Natural vaginal lubrication occurs when you are sexually excited, and when you are wet, bruising is less likely to occur. Not only is foreplay enjoyable, it serves a very real purpose!

I suffered from cystitis for about 20 years, on and off. It began on honeymoon, probably because I wasn't prepared (psychologically and physically) for intercourse. My marriage was somewhat lacking and my husband and I eventually divorced. I've remarried and have had no recurrence in the last 15 years. I'm sure that's because I now have a loving partner who knows how to arouse me fully before intercourse and with whom I can be relaxed.

When I had a relationship with a woman I don't remember having cystitis at all. Sometimes the thought of sleeping with a man, especially if they've got a big penis, horrifies me – I just feel as though I'm going to be bruised all over.

Sex and the menopause

Post-menopausal women are prone to cystitis. That's because the body no longer produces high levels of oestrogen, which keeps the vaginal walls moist and stretchy. Intercourse can make the dry vaginal and urethral tissues inflamed and sore and so urinary tract infections can easily start up.

Oestrogen replacement creams applied directly inside the vagina can prevent the occurrence of sexually-related cystitis.

Sex, cystitis and diaphragms

I had a steady partner and used my diaphragm with few problems for two years. With my next partner, I wasn't so lucky. I'm sure it had something to do with the way we fitted together anatomically! When we made love, I could feel the diaphragm pressing against my bladder.

For the next two years, I suffered a lot of 'unexplained' cystitis-like symptoms. No infection was ever found, but my bladder burned and I felt the urge to pass water a lot of the time. It got to the stage when I couldn't bear to put my cap in. Eventually I threw it away and we started to use condoms. That was six years ago and I haven't had any problems since then, touch wood!

It's not a coincidence that women who use diaphragms suffer from cystitis a lot. And apparently, it's all in the fit. An ill-fitting diaphragm will press on a woman's bladder. With the diaphragm restricting it, the bladder can't be emptied properly and that's when the problems start.

In the early 1980s Dr Larrian Gillespie, a urologist working in America, carried out a study of patients complaining of cystitis. Three out of four of these patients were diaphragm users. Dr Gillespie found that the flow of urine can be restricted by as much as 40 per cent by a diaphragm. And because the diaphragm must stay in place for six hours or more (and many women keep it in place for much longer), bacteria have a great time, breeding away in the trapped urine!

But it's not all doom and gloom for diaphragm users. After her survey, Dr Gillespie came to the conclusion that it's not diaphragms *themselves* that cause cystitis. Instead, it's the way doctors are taught to fit diaphragms that makes users prone to urinary tract infections. Doctors are taught to fit women with the largest comfortable size. But no diaphragm remains tight-fitting during sexual excitation. The main function of the cap is to hold spermicide in the correct place, which is by the cervix, so a slight variation in diaphragm size won't reduce its effectiveness. On the other hand, a diaphragm that's too small can slip out of place. This goes to show that a diaphragm must be fitted very very carefully. A correctly fitting diaphragm shouldn't press on your bladder. After being fitted with smaller diaphragms (or switching birth control methods), almost every one of Dr Gillespie's cystitis-prone patients were free of infection at the end of the year.

It's not the diaphragm, it's the cream

The spermicidal cream that you smear inside a diaphragm is a strong-smelling chemical cream. These powerful chemicals can irritate the mucous membranes of the vagina and vulva and sensitize the urethra. No wonder, then, that so many cap users complain of cystitis. If you suffer an allergic reaction like this, avoid using spermicidal creams or foams altogether. Unfortunately, using a diaphragm without spermicide won't offer you much contraceptive protection, so you may have to choose another contraceptive altogether. Ask at your local family planning clinic for advice.

Devotees of diaphragms can reduce the risk of associated cystitis by always passing water after sex, and only leaving the device in for just six hours after intercourse and no longer.

A word or two about condoms

The condom is now the most popular method of contraception in the UK – couples seeming to have foresaken the Pill in its favour. There is a huge variety of condoms now available, in all colours and flavours. You can buy them from chemists, record shops, supermarkets, pubs and by mail order.

In theory, condoms are good news for cystitis sufferers. Because they are a barrier method of contraception, they help prevent bacteria passing from one partner to another during sex. They help to protect you against all kinds of venerial disease, not just AIDS. These include herpes, gonorrhoea, syphilis, chlamydia and genital warts. Condoms also offer protection against cervical cancer. But they're no substitute for good hygiene for sufferers of sexual cystitis.

Many condoms come coated with a spermicide, so for sensitive women, using condoms can cause problems similar to those caused by using spermicidal cream with a diaphragm. If you think condoms might be causing your attacks of cystitis, change to a non-spermicidally lubricated brand of condoms.

Some women react to the antioxidants in condom rubber, which can lead to cystitis-like symptoms. Those who are allergic to latex rubber can buy Allergy (hypoallergenic) condoms or Fourex skins, made from an animal membrane. Fourex are manufactured by Schmid Laboratories in America and can be obtained by mail order in most countries (see the Useful addresses section for their address). But they are not regarded as being as safe as latex condoms as a means of preventing diseases.

Female condoms, which line and protect a woman's vagina and cervix, are fairly new on the market. Research shows them to be as effective as the male condom, but they are not recommended if you are generally allergic to rubber or spermicide.

Antibiotics

It has been proved that women who suffer from sexually-related recurrent urinary tract infections benefit from taking antibiotic drugs after intercourse. American research found that women need not take these drugs continually to keep the infections at bay – just taking them after sex is enough to ward off cystitis. This, of course, is excellent news for sufferers for whom sex has become a nightmare. However, in the light of the discovery of interstitial cystitis (see Chapter 15) and the harm that antibiotics can do to the lining of the bladder in the absence of an infection, it's probably better not to rely on antibiotics if possible. It would be better to pinpoint the actual cause of the problem to prevent the symptoms starting up in the first place, than only treat the symptoms.

Checklist for sex without tears

The only real precaution I take as a matter of course is to go to the toilet before and after sexual activity. This seems to be a key factor where my bouts of cystitis are concerned.

Spontaneous sex is out of the question, but it's worth being careful as I seem to have conquered my cystitis.

I had mountains of pills and even an operation to stretch my urethra, but the single most helpful thing that I learned from my cystitis self-help group was to pass water within 15 minutes of intercourse. It worked and cystitis became a rarity!

Lots of sufferers agree there is no one cure for cystitis. What works for one woman won't automatically guarantee a cure for another. But there are a few hard and fast rules, which have been mentioned throughout this book, and sticking to these dramatically reduces the likelihood of cystitis occurring. Similarly, there are dos and don'ts concerning sex that, if adhered to, may stop you ever suffering again. Here are the ten commandments for a cystitis-free sex life!

- *Always pass water before you have sex* It's not a good idea to have sex with a full bladder (or bowel for that matter) as it could increase the pressure and chances of bruising during sexual activity.
- *When you've emptied your bladder, drink a glass of water* This means

there will be urine in the bladder for you to pass when you've finished having sex.

- *Wash before sex.*
- *Ask your partner to wash too.*
- *Avoid sexual positions that might bruise or put pressure on the urethra and bladder* This is particularly important if your cystitis is the non-bacterial kind.
- *Use plenty of lubrication* KY Jelly helps to prevent the delicate membranes around the vulva and perineum from being damaged. Bacteria can lodge in any tiny cracks in the skin and multiply rapidly.
- *Foreplay* Sexual arousal causes the vagina to secrete its own lubrication, which means bruising is far less likely to occur. So make sure you and your partner take time to get aroused.
- *Avoid using a diaphragm* They have been shown to be a cause of cystitis. It's probably worth changing contraceptive methods if your cystitis occurs after sex.
- *Always urinate immediately after having sex* This is important as surveys have shown that urinating within ten minutes of having sex can significantly improve your chances of not getting cystitis.
- *Wash after sex* Again, this helps to prevent bacteria from spreading to the urethra and bladder.

13

Alternative remedies

The one thing about cystitis that almost every woman complains of is the way it makes them feel diseased – exhausted, run down, scared; in effect, really poorly! That's because cystitis doesn't just affect the bladder and urethra, it affects your whole system. Alternative or complementary medicine, which focuses on the body as a whole rather than just the symptoms, can be used to back up treatment from your GP (and your own self-help) to put you in the pink again.

The biggest bonus with alternative remedies is that they can help when conventional medicine (such as antibiotics or surgery) is no longer effective. Sometimes, very sadly, cystitis sufferers find themselves facing an uncertain future. With the few short words, 'I'm sorry, but there's nothing more we can do for you', they find the National Health Service has, in effect, washed its hands of them. Such women must find a way to live with their cystitis. Alternative remedies, combined with the self-help practices outlined in this book, offer an answer.

In the Western world very little medical research has been done into complementary cures, and the effectiveness of alternative medicines continues to be questioned. Wherever possible, the remedies discussed in this chapter are described with accompanying recommendations from sufferers who've tried and tested them. It's worth remembering, though, that not all of these treatments will work for everybody. But if they work for you, don't keep it to yourself. Spread the word and help other sufferers too!

Important

All pregnant women should consult their doctor or ante-natal carer before trying any of the remedies suggested here.

Acupuncture

The ear and the bladder are controlled by the kidney meridian in Chinese medicine. My GP doesn't recognize a link, however. I've suffered from cystitis quite badly since 1989. Although this has almost cleared up now – I still get the odd twinge after sex when my bladder feels bruised – I developed a severe attack of labyrinthitis (a viral inflammation of the inner ear) for which I'm receiving acupuncture. I'm virtually housebound because I feel so sick and dizzy all the time, but I do feel that the acupuncture is helping.

My acupuncturist says there's an old Chinese saying that you choose your own illness, you lose the things that are the most important to you. I think she's right. With my illness I've lost my independence. I've found it very difficult to ask people to help me with the simplest things like shopping for food.

Simply defined, acupuncture is the science of puncturing the skin with needles to relieve pain. In reality, its practice is much more complicated. Acupuncture is part of traditional Chinese medicine, which respects the patient's *ch'i* (pronounced 'chee'), an invisible energy running beneath the surface of the skin that keeps the body warm and healthy. A person can become ill when the flow of *ch'i* becomes too weak or too strong or partially blocked. Acupuncturists aim to stimulate and correct the flow of *ch'i* and so restore health by inserting thin needles at particular points along the patient's body. They may also burn herbs (moxibustion) to further stimulate energy. Acupuncture is a powerful form of medicine and can be used for treating a very wide range of diseases, including cystitis.

According to acupuncture, cystitis occurs when there is cold in the body trapping heat; just becoming cold or getting your feet wet can set it off as in Chinese medicine there is a line running between the bladder and the feet. Amazingly, despite the huge difference between the Chinese and Western ways of thinking, this belief is reflected in the traditional old wives' tale: a whole generation of women avoid getting cold or wet feet because they've been warned by their mothers, and grandmothers before them, that this can cause cystitis!

I've had cystitis quite a few times in my lifetime and I've always associated it with becoming cold or damp, like getting caught in the rain. That's why I'm always careful to dry my feet really well whenever they get wet!

Also in Chinese medicine there is a line connecting the heart, small intestine and bladder, so practitioners say that cystitis can often occur when you are emotionally vulnerable. In fact, many women do suffer from cystitis at times of emotional stress, although they rarely link the two. Practitioners of Chinese medicine believe that health is a state of total harmony between the physical, emotional and spiritual aspects of the individual. Many things can upset this balance – emotionally important states, such as worry, anger and grief. Each of these emotions has a particular effect on the body's energy balance and leads to disease, in the widest sense of the word. Fear seems to be the emotion that triggers cystitis.

If you find it hard to believe that your symptoms are created by your emotional state, just stop and think about it for a minute. It's widely known that people suffering fright wet their pants, and emotionally distressed children often wet the bed. Feeling down can trigger digestive and, thence, bowel and urinary problems, so it's not surprising that a long standing or recurring background fear can cause pretty strong cystitis symptoms.

I never noticed the link between how I felt emotionally and my physical health more strongly than the time I had a massive row with my mother. We really came to blows and I thought for a while that our relationship would never recover. At the same time I felt like I was getting cystitis – nothing serious enough to go to the doctors about, but uncomfortable enough to remind me of the emotional pain I'm sure we were both suffering.

Acupuncture helps energize the body to resist fear and so may be very effective in treating cystitis. It also seems to help in treating gynaecological problems, including irregular periods, repeated miscarriages, hot flushes and premenstrual tension. Contact the Council for Acupuncture, the British Acupuncture Association or the Traditional Acupuncture Society (Useful addresses section at the back of the book) for a list of registered practitioners in your area.

Homeopathy

I had an appalling period of 12 to 18 months of continuous bouts of cystitis. This culminated in the most miserable New Year's Day, which I spent wallowing in the bath, sick with pain and miserable with discomfort. I had, rather uncharacteristically, got quite drunk the previous night. Fed up with taking antibiotics, I contacted a homeopath.

She took a long, detailed history and decided that the most vulnerable, weakest part of my body was my sexual and reproductive organs. Because I didn't actually have the symptoms of cystitis when I saw her, the homeopath gave me a constitutional prescription to build up my health and prevent a recurrence. She also suggested giving up red wine and coffee and recommended that I stop using my contraceptive cap, explaining that 90 per cent of cases were aggravated by one or more of these three things.

I was so desperate to put an end to my suffering that I did all that she recommended. I stopped drinking coffee and red wine completely for about six months and threw away my cap. To my absolute amazement I have not had any subsequent attacks. I've changed nothing else in my life and I've never had cystitis since, even though I now drink coffee and red wine again in moderation. I don't suppose I'll ever know whether it was red wine, coffee or my cap that was causing the problem, but I don't mind. All I care about is that I seem to have beaten it.

My mum gets cystitis all the time, but won't explore the alternative medicine route. Instead she's agreed with her GP to try taking antibiotics for a year in an effort to get rid of it. She's six months in and still suffering. I feel we are very similar, which makes me even more grateful to my homeopath. If I hadn't gone to see her about my cystitis, I'm sure I'd still be plagued with it.

Homeopathy was 'invented' in 1790 by Samuel Hahnemann, a German doctor. In contrast to orthodox medicine, homeopathy sees symptoms as positive attempts by the body to rid itself of the disease. Working on the principle that 'like cures like', homeopathic treatments encourage the body to fight disease. By giving a remedy that in a healthy person is capable of producing similar symptoms to those being suffered by the patient stimulates the body's natural defences to resist the infection. Thus, homeopathy stimulates the body to release its own healing powers. Initially, therefore, the symptoms of the illness may well worsen, but well-being increases as the treatment is continued.

Before a diagnosis is made, the homeopath will want to examine your medical history in depth. Great emphasis is placed on lifestyle, diet and general health, and your personality and emotional disposition will also be taken into account. Cystitis is reported to respond very well to homeopathic treatment as sufferers can be very precise about their symptoms. Pinpointing the exact source of the discomfort helps the homeopath build up a clear picture of the patient's underlying illness.

As each individual has their own weaknesses, it is almost impossible to talk about routine homeopathic 'cures'. There are, however, a few remedies that tend to work well in relieving acute cystitis for most women. Cantharis helps with burning pains, while Pulsatilla helps relieve the kind of cystitis that has milder pains that worsen when you're lying on your back. Sasparilla can relieve the shooting pain a cystitis sufferer feels at the end of urination. And Aconite can work well if taken at the first signs of cystitis, especially if there's a chill involved – it can also nip a cold in the bud!

Not only does homeopathy have a high success rate in treating acute cystitis, it can also help get rid of the underlying weaknesses that encourage recurrent attacks. Preventative homeopathic treatments are called *Constitutional remedies*. Staphisagria, for example, can be prescribed constitutionally for women whose cystitis is typically associated with sex. Constitutional remedies can only be prescribed by a qualified homeopath once they have built up a clear picture of your emotional and physical health.

I was very sceptical about the effectiveness of homeopathy and natural medicine, but being seven miles from the doctors I had to try something first. Now, I always take homeopathic Cantharis at the first signs of urgency.

Homeopathic medicine is now sometimes available in the UK on the National Health Service. There are five homeopathic hospitals (London, Glasgow, Liverpool, Bristol and Tunbridge Wells), as well as numerous homeopathic clinics. To find a good homeopath, consult the register held by the Society of Homeopaths (for their address, see the Useful addresses section at the back of the book, enclosing a stamped addressed envelope when you write if you'd like them to send you a full list of homeopaths).

You can learn to use some homeopathic remedies at home as short courses outlining the basics of homeopathy are often given at natural health centres. In the UK, homeopathic medicines are available over the counter at chemists or by post from several pharmacies (see the Useful addresses section for companies that make or supply a full range of homeopathic medicines and despatch them by mail order).

If you decide to try acute remedies (e.g. Sasparilla, Aconite and Staphisagria) you must take them at the first signs of an attack. If a remedy is going to work for you (and you haven't taken any coffee or eucalyptus oil, which negate the effects of homeopathy), it will usually take effect immediately if it is well matched to your symptoms, so you would be wise to visit your GP if symptoms continue.

Herbal medicine

People have used herbs for thousands of years to prevent and cure diseases – in fact, herbalism is the oldest form of medicine known to mankind. Our ancestors, by trial and error, found the most effective local plants to heal their illnesses. Although herbalism is still classed as an alternative or complementary form of medicine, it is still the most widely practised form worldwide, with over 80 per cent of the world's population relying on herbs for health.

Chinese herbalism uses herbs, in conjunction with the principles of acupuncture, for example using 'hot' herbs to treat 'cold' conditions. Western herbalism, however, is more like orthodox medicine, with remedies being prepared to fight the prevailing symptoms. However, unlike many orthodox doctors, herbalists generally take a holistic approach to illness and always look for the underlying cause of the condition.

The healing effects of herbal remedies may be slower than those of synthetic drugs but they may ultimately be more effective. Derived from plants, they form an 'active' or 'living' medicine. Most herbs are toxic in large doses or if they are used over a long period of time, so take care.

The National Institute of Medical Herbalists, the oldest professional organization of herbal practitioners, believes that herbal medicine is particularly suited to the treatment of cystitis for two reasons. First, herbalists approach all conditions by strengthening the body so that it is less likely to suffer from any form of infection. Second, herbal treatments contain a large number of urinary antiseptics. These reduce the severity of the attacks whilst the body is strengthened to heal itself.

A few herbal remedies known to be effective in treating cystitis are described below and you may have some success with them yourself. If you want to explore the use of herbs, a properly qualified herbalist will be able to help you. Contact the National Institute of Medical Herbalists at the address given in the Useful addresses section at the back of the book for a full list of practitioners.

Alfalfa, oatstraw and cornsilk herbal teas

Two to three cups of alfalfa and oatstraw herbal teas, and one cup of cornsilk herbal tea can help prevent cystitis if you feel an attack coming on. Buy the teas already prepared or make your own infusions using the dried plants. Apparently, one cup of each a day keeps cystitis at bay! These teas are worth exploring as a long-term preventative measure.

Comfrey

Comfrey, also known as the healing herb, has many properties and uses that are often suggested by its various common names. It is called bruisewort and it's an astringent, so it can mend inflamed tissues, it is called knitback and is a pain reliever and soother, can stem an excessive flow of (menstrual) blood and heal wounds, and it is called gum plant and it makes an excellent gargle and mouthwash for throat inflammations, hoarseness and bleeding gums.

I have found that comfrey tablets are extremely good at treating cystitis, but recently found out that they have been withdrawn from health shops due to some misguided idea that they cause cancer. I believe that there is a move afoot to have them reinstated. Now I have to rely on comfrey tea, which, thankfully, is still available, and also the homeopathic comfrey made by Weleda, which goes under its Latin name of Symphytum.

I found out about this cure when someone gave me a book that mentioned comfrey as a cure for all ills. It has anti-inflammatory properties so I thought it would be effective against cystitis.

Calendula

Calendula tincture can be bought from homeopathic chemists, herbalists and good healthfood stores (also see the addresses in the Useful addresses section at the back of the book for mail order companies). Ten drops in your bath will help reduce inflammation and clear infection. Calendula ointment applied externally to the urethra and vulva can also be very soothing during a cystitis attack.

Parsley

Parsley is supposed to be good as a preventative measure for recurrent cystitis sufferers. Eat it with your salads or make an infusion from dried parsely and drink as a tea.

Juniper

Juniper is known for its antiseptic and diuretic qualities, and for its effectiveness in ridding the body of wind. Juniper is normally taken internally by eating the berries or making a tea from them. Juniper oil, derived from the berries, can irritate the skin, so use it with care. Also, in large doses, juniper can irritate the kidneys and urinary passages, so it is not recommended for those with kidney problems or if you are pregnant.

At 29, a sudden love affair brought on cystitis. One lot of antibiotics had finished and I was bleeding a little from the bladder. Unfortunately, at the time I was about to perform a matinée of the local pantomine, followed by the final performance, followed by a rock concert later. What to do? There was no time to visit the doctor and the chemist was closed. But I remembered that juniper tea had been a help in the past, so I bought some juniper berries from the local healthfood store. Over the next eight hours, I ate about 3 ounces of them and the condition improved.

My neighbour, who recovered from cancer of the bladder, had

symptoms similar to cystitis from the chemotherapy. He was helped greatly by strong juniper tea at my suggestion. I also gave crushed juniper to my ancient red setter dog to assist with his incontinence – I also gave him raw garlic which undoubtedly works for cystitis if you and your family can stand it!

Nowadays, I take a few juniper berries at the first sign of cystitis. Juniper is also very helpful for period pains and excessive menstrual bleeding.

Antitis tablets

There's a herbal remedy you can buy in tablet form at chemists and in good healthfood shops that is designed specifically to combat cystitis. The main ingredient, uva-ursi, has urinary antiseptic properties, but all the herbs contained in these tablets, known as Potter's Antitis tablets, have a diuretic action. They are available from healthfood shops and high street pharmacies or you can order them direct from (see the Useful addresses section at the back of the book for their address).

Aromatherapy and essential oils

Many women use aromatherapy to treat all kinds of different complaints – from insect bites to dandruff. This involves a mixture of aromas, massage and medicine and uses essential oils extracted from plants, flowers and herbs.

Aromatherapy can help relieve an attack of cystitis or nip one in the bud, but how does it work? Our sense of smell, as it is so closely linked with our emotions, is the key to its healing power. Further, massage encourages the body's own healing potential. It relaxes and soothes the body by relieving tension and encouraging the release of pent-up emotions. Massage can also increase your 'feel-good factor'. That's because it stimulates the release of hormones known as *endorphins*. These are the body's own painkillers, relaxants and anti-depressants.

In her book *Aromatherapy for Women* (Thorsons, 1990), Maggie Tisserand recommends several essential oil treatments for cystitis sufferers. Juniper oil may be taken in water sweetened with a little honey, and sandalwood oil can be rubbed around where the kidneys are in the lower back. She also recommends taking a lavender sitz bath. If this isn't practical, you can make up a bottle of lavender water (that's one to three drops of oil mixed with 100ml of bottled or cooled boiled water). Apply a cotton wool pad (or sanitary towel) soaked with lavender water to the vulva after each visit to the toilet.

If you'd like to try aromatherapy, contact the International Federation of Aromatherapists at the address given in the Useful addresses section at the back of the book for a full list of qualified practitioners.

Reflexology

Reflexology involves the ancient art of foot massage. A very old therapy from the Far East, reflexology works on the principle that your feet contain thousands of nerve endings, which are all connected to other parts of the body. Certain areas of the soles of the feet, therefore, represent and correspond to various parts of your body. That's why when your bladder is inflamed, the corresponding point on the soles of your feet (it's just over half-way down, on the inner arch – press it and see) may be painful and sore to the touch.

A reflexologist will massage the area to stimulate the bladder and help it to heal. Many natural therapists use reflexology as part of their basic treatment and the treatment is also often offered at beauty salons and health clubs. To find a professional reflexologist in your area contact the British School of Reflexology at the address given in the Useful addresses section.

Osteopathy

If you think osteopaths only treat people with back trouble, think again! Osteopaths aim to restore your whole body's natural balance. They gently massage, manipulate and stretch muscles that have become displaced or strained. That's why osteopathy can help women whose cystitis is due to a mildly misplaced womb and/or bladders. A combination of osteopathy and special exercises may be a welcome alternative to surgery.

There isn't a statutory register of British osteopaths and some people call themselves osteopaths after little or no formal training. The College of Osteopaths, though, is a professional organization, the members of which have passed lengthy and stringent examinations. A full list of its members can be obtained from the College at the address given in the Useful addresses section at the back of the book.

Self-help

There are lots of different treatments that can be used at home to cure and prevent attacks of cystitis. Some of the ones already described are juniper, lavender and sandalwood essential oils, which can be purchased from healthfood shops and large department stores; herbs, which can be purchased fresh or dried from healthfood shops and/or grocers, grown in your garden or growing wild on common land; and of course you can effect an enormous change in your health simply by changing your diet and hygiene habits (see Chapters 6 and 12). Listed below are a few other ways in which you can make yourself more comfortable during an attack of cystitis and, maybe, even cure it!

Garlic

Eating lots of raw, crushed garlic can help with a candida-related cystitis problem (see Chapter 5). It is a powerful antifungal plant, but it is also a strong antibiotic. Used locally (that is, inserted into the vagina) garlic cloves can fight bacterial cystitis or kill vaginal thrush, which can irritate the urethra and trigger off a cystitis attack.

> I have suffered from cystitis since I was about 11. I'm now 22 and have tried everything. I suffered attacks about every five weeks and I've missed school and work and had holidays abroad ruined because of it. Potassium citrate was a good remedy, which usually worked in 24 hours, but the best cure I've found is garlic!
> I peel a garlic clove, prick it a few times and then (I know this sounds horrible) insert it into my vagina. Somehow the vapour acts on it immediately and it usually only takes two or three hours to clear up. My step-mun told me about this when I was 18 and since then I've always used this remedy and it always works. I know it's not a pleasant remedy and garlic is a very strong smell, but when your cystitis is so bad that you can't leave the bathroom you really don't care.

Sitz baths

A sitz bath is a very shallow or 'hip' bath. Add herbs or essential oils to a small amount of lukewarm water (cold water is better if you can bear it), then sit in the bath with your knees apart. Wash your anus beforehand. Using the bottle method and urinating after your sitz bath will reduce the risk of infection from germs floating into the urethra. Open your vagina by gently inserting a finger or two, pulling down slightly to allow the water to run in. Or try placing two large plastic bowls in your bath, one filled with very hot water, the other with cold, even iced, water. Spend an alternate five minutes sitting in each. Regular sitz baths will help tone the delicate tissues of your sexual and reproductive organs and so promote healing.

Yoga

If you could only choose one form of exercise to keep your body in perfect general health, yoga should be the one you go for. Forget step classes and exercise machines at expensive gym clubs because once you've learnt the basics of yoga, you can do it for free any time, almost anywhere. All you need is a quiet room and a blanket!

There are several different forms of yoga, but all are based on improving your breathing to increase the flow of oxygen to the body and stretching your body to improve its suppleness. Yoga is generally done very slowly with a focus on meditative movement, so it is very relaxing. Studies have proved that by renewing the body, focusing the mind and stilling the emotions, yoga can reduce high blood pressure and stress, increase the suppleness of the joints and improve hormonal functioning. It can also help women who suffer from prolonged and recurrent bouts of cystitis.

Classes are often offered at alternative health centres and your local educational authority will probably run yoga day or night classes.

I suffer a lot from cystitis and one of the most useful methods of help, as I practise yoga, is to sit in the tailor pose (bend your legs at the knee, soles of the feet together). This stretches out the affected parts and certainly stops everything feeling so tight. Yoga is generally very good for a lot of women's ailments.

Some final points

Natural remedies can be very potent. If one is going to work for you, it will have done so within a week. Unless otherwise directed, it is best to use these treatments at the first signs of an infection and to continue to do so for the next seven days. If, after this time, you still think you have an infection, it's worth reassessing your problem. Perhaps it's time to consult your doctor.

Chapter 16 contains detailed case studies, many from women who have suffered very badly from cystitis for a number of years. Almost all of these women have found ways of coping with it themselves *alongside* the cures prescribed by the medical profession. Through trial and error they've had to discover what works for them. Hopefully you will find their experiences useful.

14

Other problems: when cystitis is not cystitis

I thought I'd got cystitis again. Every time I went to the loo it stung like crazy. In between times it wasn't really painful, though the whole area felt very sore. I convinced myself that I had a milder version of cystitis and tried to drink the pain away. It didn't work. No wonder! Unbeknown to me I was suffering my first attack of herpes.

I was hitchhiking back to Manchester when I developed a cystitis-like feeling. I wanted to go to the loo all the time. I sat in strangers' cars in agony trying to pretend everything was OK. Eventually I got to my doctor who took one look at me and sent me off to the special clinic. I didn't have ordinary common or garden cystitis – I'd caught gonorrhoea from my two-timing boyfriend!

The surest sign that an attack of cystitis is on its way is a burning pain. But that burning feeling and desperately needing to urinate are also the symptoms of several other infections. Some of these are only caught through sexual contact with an infected person. And some of them, such as gardnerella, arise naturally in the body but can still be sexually transmitted – that is, passed from partner to partner during sex. All of them require proper diagnosis and treatment, but it's best to try and avoid them occurring in the first place. *Great* sex is *healthy* sex and practising safer sex is the best way to be kind to your body and everyone else's!

There's more about safer sex at the end of this chapter, but first, here's more about the infections that are most easily confused with cystitis.

Chlamydia

Most typical symptom Cystitis.
Other symptoms Vaginal discharge, abdominal pain with fever. Note that symptoms vary a lot from person to person. Often the sufferer has no symptoms at all.
Other symptoms in men Penile discharge, pain in the testicles, pain or discharge in the rectum.

Chlamydia – or *Chlamydia trachomatis*, to give it its full medical name – can make you feel a bit like you've got cystitis. But chlamydia is a very different infection, affecting the genitals and sometimes the eyes and throat.

If you've not heard about chlamydia before, you'll be surprised to know that it's now one of the commonest sexually transmitted diseases around. When it infects the urethra and cervix, the sufferer may notice a thin vaginal discharge and/or lower abdominal pain occasionally with fever. But, more worryingly, it may cause no symptoms at all. At least four out of ten cases of chlamydia diagnosed in routine tests on women attending sexually transmitted diseases clinics show no symptoms at all. Meanwhile, the infection may have spread to the Fallopian tubes, causing pelvic inflammatory disease, which can result in ectopic pregnancy and infertility. Three quarters of the women who have three attacks or more are likely to become sterile.

Men can also be symptomless or else experience a burning pain passing urine and/or a discharge from the penis.

Both partners should always be tested for chlamydia. And if you're considering becoming pregnant, get yourself checked out for chlamydia first! It's been linked to miscarriage, ectopic pregnancy and premature delivery.

Although chlamydia was recognized as an infection as early as 1909, it's only in the last 30 years or so that it's been taken seriously by doctors and health workers. It has to be diagnosed by specialists, so if you think you might be suffering from chlamydia, visit a genito-urinary medicine clinic and ask for a test. Many cases aren't picked up by tests at all, however, as the disease can lie in hiding for many years until it's triggered off by another genital infection or by a change of partner.

Treatment is with tetracycline, an antibiotic (to be taken on an empty stomach). Pregnant women are usually given erythromycin instead, and a new drug called azithromycin, taken in a single dose, is being tested on men with promising results.

Like all sexually transmitted diseases, the best way to avoid it is to practise safer sex and use a condom.

Herpes

Most typical symptom For women suffering from their first attack, this is usually pain on passing urine.
Other symptoms Stinging, tingling or itching in the genital area, flu-like symptoms, temperature, pain down the thighs and legs.

Herpes are cold sores, which look like blisters or small bumps. In women these are typically found in and around the vagina, so passing urine can be terribly painful if any drips or splashes come into contact with the sores.

It's quite possible to mistake this sensation for the symptoms of cystitis, particularly if you are suffering from your first ever attack and/or if the sores are inside the vagina and not visible. If you don't feel the need to urinate frequently, however, you can be sure you don't have cystitis!

Herpes are nearly always transmitted sexually. The blisters are caused by the virus, herpes simplex virus II, similar to the type that produces cold sores or blisters around the mouth and nose. They are normally painful, especially if they burst to leave a small red ulcer. These usually heal within a week or two, although it may take a month for an attack to clear up.

When the sores disappear, the virus enters a latent state, when it is no longer contagious. A new attack can occur at any time and there is no limit to the number of attacks a herpes sufferer may experience, although, for many people, the first attack is the worst. Usually symptoms become milder and clear up more quickly with each attack. About half the people who get one attack of herpes never have another one.

As yet, there is no known cure for herpes. The symptoms can be relieved with sulpha creams and corticosteroids. Wearing loose cotton clothing and underwear during an attack helps. Try to keep the area cool and dry.

It has been suggested that there is a strong link between herpes and cancer of the cervix, but this has not actually been proved. However, women who suffer from herpes should have frequent cervical smear tests, preferably every 6 to 12 months.

Gonorrhoea

Most typical symptom Pain on passing urine.
Other symptoms Vaginal discharge, abdominal pain, fever backache.
Other symptoms in men Penile discharge, or discharge in the rectum.

One of the main symptoms of gonorrhoea in women is pain on passing water. That is if it gives rise to any symptoms at all, because women with gonorrhoea rarely show any symptoms until its irreparable damage has been done. Left untreated, gonorrhoea can infect and inflame the Fallopian tubes (the tubes that carry eggs from the ovaries to the womb), causing scarring, blockages and infertility.

Thankfully, the incidence of gonorrhoea has fallen dramatically since the mid 1980s, partly because of the increased use of condoms resulting from AIDS awareness. In the UK, the incidence of gonorrhoea fell by almost 60 per cent between 1985 and 1988 and it still appears to be on the decline. Gonorrhoea is still considered to be a very serious disease, however, because of the complications it causes if left untreated. And it has been found to go very much hand in hand with chlamydia. So, all those who test positive for gonorrhoea should also be tested for chlamydia, which, if present, will require different treatment.

Gonorrhoea can only be transmitted sexually. It is caught by having intercourse or intimate contact with an infected person. This is because the bacterium that causes the disease – the gonococcus – cannot survive for any length of time away from the body. It's possible to develop gonorrhoea in the throat if you have oral sex with an infected person. Occasionally sufferers may infect their own eyes.

Men almost always know when they have gonorrhoea, usually some two to five days after contracting it. At first, there is a burning sensation on passing urine. This is then followed by a penile discharge of yellow pus as the disease begins to affect the urethra. In women, the most common site of early, uncomplicated gonorrhoea is the cervix, so there may be cervical discharge. The urethra may also be affected. But even in cases where both the urethra *and* cervix are involved, there may still be no warning signs of infection.

Sometimes, small abscesses form around the external opening of the urethra. When the inflammation spreads along the urethra to the base of the bladder, it will cause cystitis-like symptoms. Sufferers will experience a frequent urge to urinate, although there may be only a small amount of water to pass. What little there is burns very badly.

Gonorrhoea is best treated at a special clinic (see page 54). It can be treated effectively – usually with large doses of penicillin – if it is caught early enough. If you think that you might have been exposed to the infection – even if you have no symptoms at all – go to a special clinic and ask to be checked out.

Gardnerella or bacterial vaginosis

Most typical symptom Itchy, fishy-smelling discharge.
Other symptoms Burning cystitis-like sensation.

Gardnerella vaginalis is a strain of anaerobic bacteria which infects the vaginal secretions rather than the walls of the vagina itself. Like most vaginitis, it occurs when the vagina's delicately balanced flora is upset. Present in every healthy vagina, gardnerella is only troublesome if conditions here become too alkaline, which means it multiplies out of all proportion. Gardnerella, often referred to as bacterial vaginosis, may be triggered by overwashing or douching, using perfumed soap and deodorants or even having a period (blood is alkaline and so periods of prolonged bleeding can often cause gardnerella to occur).

The most obvious symptom of this infection is an unpleasant fishy-smelling discharge. Like thrush, gardnerella is very itchy but gardnerella produces a thin, white or grey vaginal discharge whereas a thrush discharge is thick and curd-like. This discharge may irritate the urethra and give rise to apparent cystitis-like symptoms so it could be confused with a urinary infection.

Gardnerella is very common, but left undetected and untreated, can be quite serious. It has been linked with problems during pregnancy, including recurrent miscarriages. Gardnerella can be diagnosed at a special clinic, where it is easily treated with Flagyl (metronidazole) tablets taken by mouth. Flagyl is a very powerful antibiotic with some nasty side-effects, such as severe nausea, thrush, stomach cramps and constipation. If you have to take more than one course of Flagyl, you should wait at least six weeks before beginning the second course. Flagyl should never be taken during pregnancy or while breastfeeding, as it can be excreted in breast milk.

Women prone to thrush should ask for a course of thrush treatment to take at the same time. Flagyl also kills off some white blood cells, so it shouldn't be taken by anyone with blood diseases or diseases of the central nervous system. It should be taken with food, rather than on an empty stomach, but never drink alcohol when you are taking a course of Flagyl.

The use of Flagyl alone may not be enough to cure and prevent attacks of anaerobic vaginal infections such as gardnerella. The trouble with anaerobic bacteria is that they thrive in oxygen-free conditions. That's one of the reasons they are so common. You can help prevent further attacks by keeping the vagina as acidic as possible. You can do this by adding a little lemon juice or vinegar to some water. These solutions should be inserted into the vagina one of the following ways:

- use a spermicide applicator or a cap or diaphragm
- dampen cotton wool balls in the solutions and insert them into the vagina in a diaphragm
- dip or soak a tampon or natural sponge in the solution, insert it into the vagina and leave in place overnight
- use yogurt on tampons and vinegar or lemon juice in the bath.

And don't forget garlic, a powerful antibiotic which has been used by women for centuries to treat vaginal infections. Inserting a peeled, pricked garlic clove into the vagina may help cure an attack of gardnerella.

Non-specific vaginitis/urethritis (NSU)

Most typical symptoms Burning sensation on passing urine.
Other symptoms Infective, vaginal discharge/cervicitis with pus.
Symptoms in men Infective (pussy) discharge from the penis.

In the simplest terms, NSU means you have bacterial urethritis. It is a very common sexually transmitted disease and has far outstripped gonorrhoea in incidence. About 50 per cent of NSU is caused by chlamydia. Other cases are caused by *Ureaplasma urealyticum, Trichomonas vaginalis,* Herpes simplex and genital warts, but many cases remain unexplained.

After a urine culture has been made from a urine sample and a swab from the urethra/vagina has been examined, the organism causing the urethritis can be identified and the patient will be rediagnosed accordingly. For example, if a patient complains of cystitis-like symptoms but is found to have chlamydia, they will be described as suffering from chlamydial NSU. But while in men unexplained urethritis would continue to be described as NSU, women displaying the same symptoms would be described as having a non-specific genital infection or non-specific vaginitis.

Men suffering from NSU will almost certainly have acquired this sexually. Symptoms usually appear two to six weeks after they have come into contact with an infected partner, although the incubation period can be as short as one week. The main symptoms are pain and difficulty passing urine (but usually not increased frequency) and urethral discharge, most noticeable on first emptying the bladder.

Only about one in four women have any symptoms of NSU, which, when they do occur, are an increased vaginal discharge and some pain and difficulty on passing urine. They may also have cervicitis (an inflamed or reddened cervix), together with an unusually heavy, white or yellow discharge. Sometimes this is streaked with blood. The vagina may be sore and itchy. Most women are diagnosed on the basis of contact with a man with NSU or as a result of routine screening for chlamydia or investigation for pelvic inflammatory disease (PID).

One of the main problems with NSU is that it's unaffected by many antibiotics routinely used in general pratice – penicillins, co-trimoxazole, trimethoprim and ciprofloxacin. Worse still, sometimes symptoms appear to improve when treated with these drugs, which lulls the patient, and doctor, into a false sense of security. Their hopes are then dashed when the symptoms return or, even worse, when complications develop.

NSU must always be treated as soon as possible as it can have complications. Epididymo-orchitis is the commonest complication in men, which is painful, swollen testicles. Reiter's syndrome is a rare but serious complication, which includes eye inflammation and arthritis. Fortunately, Reiter's syndrome only affects 1 per cent of men with NSU. Pelvic infection is by far the most common complication in women. This can affect a woman's fertility, so it must be diagnosed and treated as soon as possible (there's more about PID later in this chapter).

NSU should be treated with tetracycline or erythromycin (the latter is suitable for pregnant women). It's important for patients to avoid sex until they've been given the all clear. Non-specific vaginitis can also be treated locally. If the infection is bacterial, a sulpha cream, such as Sultrin or Vagitrol, will be prescribed. If no bacteria are found, the infection will probably be treated with tetracycline. It is advisable not to have intercourse during treatment and, possibly, to abstain for a short while afterwards to allow the tissues to heal properly.

If you've read the early part of this book, or even the early part of this chapter, you'll know that good vaginal health relies on the vagina's natural secretions remaining acidic rather than alkaline as the acidity keeps potentially harmful organisms in check. Non-specific vaginitis is no different. It attacks the vagina when the secretions become too alkaline, allowing various bacteria to multiply to nuisance levels. And, as with bacterial cystitis, non-specific vaginitis need not be acquired sexually, but can arise when germs that live happily in other parts of the body, but not in the vagina, find their way there. Help prevent non-specific vaginitis, and cystitis of course, by always wiping away from the urethra and by washing after a bowel movement and before and after sex.

Pelvic inflammatory disease (PID)

Most typical symptoms Acute abdominal pain.
Other symptoms Backache, painful intercourse, cystitis-like symptoms.

Pelvic inflammatory disease is the name given to describe one or more related infections of the ovaries, Fallopian tubes and womb. PID can be caused by bacteria arising naturally within the body, perhaps triggered off by the use of an IUD or an abortion. But it can also be caused by sexually transmitted bacteria, such as those that cause gonorrhoea and chlamydia.

Not all women will experience PID in the same way. Most commonly, only the Fallopian tubes are affected (salpingitis), but the ovaries may be affected (oophoritis), sometimes both the ovaries and the tubes (salpingo-oophoritis) and/or the uterus (endometritis). This is why symptoms vary so much. They range from sudden, very intense abdominal pain with a high temperature, to nagging backache or leg pain, painful intercourse with bleeding and painful or irregular periods. Worryingly, symptoms are often so mild that women hardly notice them. But an increased frequency of urination, burning on or an inability to empty the bladder when urinating are symptoms of PID that could easily be mistaken for cystitis.

PID is a serious disease and must be diagnosed and treated properly. The best place to go is to a genito-urinary clinic, where a wider range of tests is available as they specialize in this area of medicine and you will probably get quicker and more accurate results. To avoid reinfection it's important that your partner gets seen too. Even though your partner may have no symptoms, they could be harbouring PID-causing bacteria.

PID is treated with antibiotics, preferably the one effective in conquering the particular organism causing the problem (if it can be identified). Treated early enough, pelvic infections often clear up quickly. More serious cases may take longer though, and severely affected tissue may have to be surgically removed. As with all illness, get plenty of rest, build up the body's immune system with a good diet and avoid physical and mental stress, which weaken the body's natural defences to disease. Look after yourself to prevent further attacks.

Ureaplasma

Most typical symptom Urethritis in men; usually no symptoms in women.

Ureaplasma causes one in four of all NSU infections in men and the symptoms of this infection are similar to cystitis.

The infection is caused by a sexually transmitted infection called *Ureaplasma urealyticum* (also called *T-mycoplasma*). It is now so commonplace (it is often found in the genital tracts of apparently healthy people who have no symptoms of infection) that many genito-urinary laboratories can't afford to test for them, although they recognize its significance in causing urethritis and cystitis.

Ureasplasma is often found with chlamydia and, like chlamydia, it often gives rise to no symptoms at all. Ureaplasma can cause cervicitis or PID in women, which in turn gives rise to cystitis-like symptoms. If you have suffered from unexplained bouts of cystitis or PID, make sure you are screened for this organism. Ureaplasma is treated with tetracycline (or erythromycin) antibiotics, although some strains resist treatment and a follow-up check about a month later is recommended.

Trichomoniasis

Most typical symptom A thin, foamy, white or greenish-yellow, smelly discharge.
Other symptoms Burning sensation when passing urine, sore, swollen

vagina. Men often have no symptoms but can be carrying the infection.

Trichomoniasis (commonly known as 'trich' or 'TV') is a vaginal infection that can also cause apparent cystitis-like symptoms. It's far less common today than it used to be. In 1983, sexually transmitted diseases clinics saw a total of 18,300 new cases whereas ten years later, in 1993, this figure had fallen to just 5300. Doctors don't know what's caused this downturn in the incidence of trichomoniasis, but one possible reason could be a general improvement in both personal and public hygiene (trichomoniasis is the one infection that it is actually possible to catch from a toilet seat!).

The infection is caused by the parasite *Trichomonas vaginalis*, a tiny, one-celled organism that feeds on other cells. The organism survives in warm, moist environments.

In some women, it is a normal and harmless inhabitant of the vagina and bladder. When too many of them are present, an infection will flare up and the vagina and vulva become swollen and sore. Women with trichomoniasis will usually notice a thin and foamy discharge, which may be white or greenish-yellow in colour and excessively smelly. If the urethra and bladder become infected as well, or just irritated by the discharge, you'll feel as though you've got cystitis and you'll probably feel a burning sensation when passing urine.

Both men and women can suffer from trichomoniasis and it can be sexually transmitted. The *Trichomonas* parasite can survive for a few hours outside the body, so it's possible to become infected from moist towels and wash cloths and even saunas and swimming pools.

It's easier to detect trichomoniasis in women as the symptoms are more immediate. The parasite can be identified in urine, but the normal procedure carried out at health clinics is to use a 'wet mount'. Some of the vaginal discharge is placed on a glass slide with a saline solution where the *Trichomonas* parasites can be seen swimming about with their whip-like tentacles.

Trichomoniasis is treated with Flagyl antibiotics. Help prevent further attacks of trichomoniasis by keeping the vagina as acidic as possible. The self-help remedies that help keep gardnerella at bay will be effective in preventing trichomoniasis. Always remember to get your sexual partner treated as they may be infected too.

Urinary incontinence

Most typical symptom Loss of control over the bladder – simply leaking when you don't expect or want to! This is what doctor's call 'involuntary loss of urine'.

Cystitis sufferers often lose control over their bladders during a full-blown attack, but many women become incontinent at some point in their lives for lots of other reasons.

An amazing 8 per cent of the general population suffer from incontinence, but there isn't a single, universally accepted definition of this condition. Most doctors would only describe a patient as *incontinent* when their loss of urine is so involuntary or occurs so often that it has become a social problem. Anyone who suffers from severe incontinence will know how it can affect every part of life. Apart from the obvious problem of becoming sore from wet underwear, a sex life and relationship may also suffer. In fact, the more severe the incontinence problem, the more life-changing the consequences will be.

Many women accept that a small amount of urine will leak out if they sneeze unexpectedly. And there must be plenty of people who do aerobics who dread doing star jumps for the same reason. In fact, a small degree of incontinence is very common in most women. Experts say one in three women aged between 25 and 55 suffer from *stress incontinence* – that's when urine leaks out of the bladder during exercise, coughing, laughing, sneezing or just a very full bladder. This is often the result of childbirth, when the muscles supporting the bladder neck or urethra have been weakened by being overstretched.

Urge incontinence is more typically associated with cystitis. Indeed, as mentioned before, it is often one of the symptoms of cystitis. Urge incontinence means that you need to empty your bladder, but can't hold on long enough to make it to the toilet. This type of incontinence is also associated with a hysterectomy and other gynaecological surgery. Urinary incontinence is particularly prevalent in elderly people – older women usually suffering from a mixture of stress and urge incontinence. Urge incontinence is often caused by an overactive or 'unstable' bladder, perhaps following a stroke or other disease of the nervous system, when the brain is no longer able to send messages properly to control the bladder.

Occasionally, incontinence might be the result of having a large fibroid or a prolapsed bladder or womb. That's why you should visit your GP if you are suffering from any incontinence, whether it is with or without pain.

Incontinence is a treatable condition. The exercises described in Chapter 4 to strengthen pelvic floor muscles will help younger women to increase their bladder control. Vaginal cones are a relatively new treatment for stress incontinence and are an alternative to pelvic floor exercises. The cones come in several different weights and are best used in the privacy of your own home where you can carry out normal daily activities. At first, women use the lightest one, keeping it in the vagina for 15 minutes twice daily. As the muscles gradually strengthen, you can progress to the heavier cones. Apparently, seven out of ten users report an improvement in their pelvic floor strength. One survey (Peattie, et al.) studied 30 women who were awaiting corrective surgery for stress incontinence. It reported that 'after just one month of the exercises with the cones, 70 per cent of the women felt they were improved or cured'. After the trial, only 19 of the 30 women still wanted corrective surgery and the gynaecologists overseeing the study concluded that 'cone therapy may be as effective as surgical correction'. So, if your stress incontinence problem is getting you down, it may be time to invest in a set.

Femina cones are only available direct from Colgate Medical by mail order (see Useful addresses section at the back of the book for their address).

Urge incontinence is treated by 'retraining' the bladder. Sufferers learn to pass increasingly larger volumes of urine, leaving longer and longer intervals between doing so. The patient relearns to control the muscles that empty the bladder. Incontinent post-menopausal women may be helped by hormone replacement therapy. See your GP for more information.

Safer sex

'Safer sex' is a phrase that has been coined by health experts keen to stop the rise in sexually transmitted diseases, especially the killer HIV virus. Practising safer sex is essential to avoid contracting not only HIV, but almost all of the diseases mentioned in this chapter.

What *is* safer sex, though? Safer sex is that which minimizes the dangers. Unsafe sex is:

- anal sex, which AIDS/HIV experts consider to be very risky, even with a condom
- vaginal, anal or oral sex without a condom.

If you avoid these, you will be practising safer sex.

The use of condoms has always been recognized as a way to stop the spread of sexually transmitted diseases, but condoms have never been so easily available as they are today. No longer just stocked in chemists, condoms are a common feature in men's and women's toilets, garages, record shops and supermarkets. And condoms are given out free at family planning and sexually transmitted disease clinics.

The good thing about condoms is that they help to protect you against all kinds of venereal disease, not just AIDS. These include herpes, gonorrhoea, syphilis, chlamydia and genital warts. Condoms also offer protection against cervical cancer. Using a condom radically reduces the risks of contracting sexually transmitted diseases or passing a recurrent problem like thrush backwards and forwards between partners. As many infections, such as thrush, irritate the urethra and can actually cause urethritis, safer sex makes sense for cystitis sufferers too!

15
Interstitial cystitis

Another time when cystitis is not cystitis is when it is interstitial cystitis, a little-known bladder complaint the symptoms of which are very similar to those of cystitis. Confused? Don't worry, this chapter asks questions and finds answers to throw more light on the matter.

Is interstitial cystitis an infection?

No. Unlike cystitis, which is often caused by the presence of bacteria in the bladder, interstitial cystitis is an *inflammation* of the bladder's lining.

Is that the main difference between the two then?

Yes. The two conditions affect the body differently in the long term, but the main difference between interstitial cystitis and cystitis is that the latter is commonly an inflammation of the bladder due to bacterial *infection*. Interstitial cystitis is *not* an infection and is not caused by germs.

But the symptoms of the inflammation are very similar to those of cystitis, aren't they?

Yes, the symptoms sufferers complain of are often indistinguishable from those of true cystitis. That's why the condition is so difficult to diagnose in its early stages.

For a start, sufferers will want to go to the toilet a lot and may still feel the urge to urinate even when their bladder is empty. The pain associated with interstitial cystitis is likely to be chronic rather than acute – that's more of a nagging, dragging kind of pain rather than a sudden sharp one. None the less, it will be enough to make you feel most uncomfortable.

What causes interstitial cystitis?

The three main triggers of interstitial cystitis appear to be allergies, recurrent infections (cystitis) and antibiotics (treatment for cystitis). Allergies have been discussed in Chapter 4 as a general cause of cystitis. Unfortunately, suffering from cystitis and, consequently, being treated for it are actually the other two main *causes* of interstitial cystitis.

What? Cystitis can lead to interstitial cystitis?
How can this be so?

Well, it's all to do with the bladder and its delicate lining. The simple process of the bladder becoming inflamed – perhaps due to an allergy –

may trigger permanent cell changes in your bladder's lining. Antibiotic drugs prescribed to treat cystitis may effect a similar kind of cell change. Dr Larrian Gillespie of the University of California, Irvine, an American urologist researching this condition, found that the use of antibiotics in the absence of a bacterial infection can actually damage the bladder's inner, protective lining and so lead to interstitial cystitis.

Are all types of antibiotics bad for interstitial cystitis sufferers?

Dr Larrian Gillespie suggests that nitrofurantoin (Furadantin), a broad-spectrum antibiotic used specifically for urinary tract infection, is the main offender here.

What exactly happens to the bladder's lining?

With interstitial cystitis, the bladder becomes so inflamed that scar tissue forms all over the bladder wall, making the bladder stiff and inflexible. After a while, because it can no longer expand to its normal capacity, the pressure of just the smallest amount of fluid in the bladder makes sufferers feel decidedly 'uncomfortable'. Someone with interstitial cystitis will frequently feel the urge to empty their bladder. Although some sufferers say they have to urinate 60 or 70 times a day, a drastically reduced bladder capacity only usually occurs in the most severe of cases.

Where does interstitial cystitis come from?

The current thinking is that interstitial cystitis is an auto-immune disease – the body fighting itself! What happens is that the body detects a substance in the urine that it believes to be foreign and this sets off an auto-immune reaction. This means that antibodies are sent to the bladder, the site of the 'sensitivity', to battle against the invader. Unfortunately, as they gather to combat the enemy, they also do damage to the battle site – the lining of the bladder.

This lining has a coated surface designed to protect the delicate underlying tissues from the harmful effects of bacteria and other substances in urine. However, once this protective surface is destroyed, the underlying layers are exposed and vulnerable – a bit like a tooth without its protective enamel. These quickly become inflamed by contact with acidic urine, which causes the pain, frequency and burning sensations that accompany interstitial cystitis.

Drugs such as antibiotics and the Pill are thought to trigger the auto-immune reaction, and smoking and diet may also be factors, but researchers still don't know all the culprits for sure.

How common is interstitial cystitis?

One thing about interstitial cystitis that doctors seem certain about is that it's mainly a women's complaint – nearly 90 per cent of sufferers are female.

It used to be thought that interstitial cystitis was largely a post-menopausal disorder. Now, however, it is recognized in large numbers of women under 40 years of age. No one's certain how many sufferers there are of this complaint, but it is estimated that some 500,000 adults suffer from interstitial cystitis in the United States alone.

How do you get an accurate diagnosis?

Initially, the diagnosis of interstitial cystitis is a process of eliminating all the other infections or diseases, such as chlamydia, that could be causing your cystitis-like symptoms. Similarly, anatomical defects, bladder cancer or a kidney disorder must also be ruled out. The only way of accurately diagnosing the condition, however, is to inspect the bladder walls with a cystoscope. The bladder is distended under general anaesthetic so that the pin prick haemorrhages in the bladder wall that characterize interstitial cystitis can clearly be seen. Even in the early stages of the condition, before the bladder's capacity has been noticeably reduced, these will show up as tiny red marks.

So what should you do if you think you have interstitial cystitis?

If you have read all the questions and answers in this chapter, you will realize how important it is that you get an accurate diagnosis. Antibiotics handed out by your GP for a supposed bladder infection that turns out to be interstitial cystitis will be at best useless in effecting a cure and at worst greatly aggravate the condition.

If you suspect interstitial cystitis, you should ask your GP to refer you immediately to a urologist for further tests.

Is there a cure for interstitial cystitis?

Yes. Fortunately, there are several treatments that may help sufferers. If they don't offer a permanent cure, they at least offer relief from symptoms. Treatments for interstitial cystitis include:

- *dimethyl sulphoxide* or DMSO for short, which is an anti-inflammatory agent that also dilates the blood vessels, providing pain relief in 70 to 80 per cent of the women who use it
- *elmiron* a substance that coats the inflamed bladder wall, helping to provide a protective lining and so preventing 'acid burn' from the urine

- *stretching the bladder* which can help by breaking up the existing scar tissue.

Can anyone else help?

As yet, there isn't an interstitial cystitis association in the UK and most of the research being done is in the USA. The Women's Health Information Centre in London keep up-to-date information on all aspects of women's health and so may be able to give you more information as and when they receive it. Write to them (enclosing a stamped, self-addressed envelope) or call in for more information at the address given in the Useful addresses section at the back of the book.

16

Some case studies

All the cases here are very different and have been chosen to show the wide range of causes, severity and problems of cystitis.

Susan Shepherd suffered from the emotional effects of recurrent cystitis until she visited a herbalist. After changing her diet and taking many self-help steps to prevent further attacks, Susan has now broken her cystitis pattern and feels in control of her own body.

I've suffered from cystitis for the last three years. It started about 18 months after I had a hysterectomy, with bouts of the dreaded affliction occurring at least once a month.

I felt desperate when I suffered badly, became very depressed and morbid and particularly isolated. I wasn't too worried when the cystitis first started. I'd had the occasional attack every now and then over the last 20 years, but when I was still suffering 6 months on, I knew then that this was something different. I felt very stressed and, although I'm only 42, I felt really old. I couldn't believe I had a chronic illness and worried that I might have to put up with it for the rest of my life.

I tried conventional medicine, but the male doctors were absolutely hopeless. They really didn't listen when I told them my cystitis was seriously interfering with my professional career. I realized afterwards that this was the wrong thing to say. Men in their position usually think a woman's career isn't important. Anyway, I decided to try a different tack. When I next saw my urologist, I said my cystitis was so bad, I couldn't be a 'good wife'. I had to practise this one a lot to myself before I could say it convincingly and without a smile on my face. But it paid off because then they started listening to me!

I had an operation to stretch the neck of my bladder and urethra, which didn't work – I still kept getting cystitis. Finally, my urologist told me that there was nothing more they could do for me. So I've had to look, not for a cure, but for ways to cope with it and prevent it occurring again.

As my GP had admitted he couldn't help me, I decided to consult a herbalist. I found her number in my local phone book. I'd read about this sort of medicine in my library books, but I think I struck lucky really. From my first visit I thought I could be cured. This helped me to live with it. It's not cheap, though, and I have spent a lot of money, which I don't begrudge.

My herbalist advised a radical change in my diet and diagnosed candida – thrush throughout the body. I attempted to eliminate all foods containing yeast and sugar. She also advised abstinence from strawberries and tomatoes and no more tea or coffee. It was all very spartan. Nevertheless, the symptoms persisted and if I weakened and had a glass of wine or ate chocolate, a severe bout usually followed. So, I never left the house without a packet of bicarbonate of soda, lemon barley water and a bottle of herbal medicine.

For the last three months, I've been cystitis-free and the quality of my life has improved immeasurably. But I'm constantly on my guard against further attacks and do all I can to avoid them. I work in a university, which is, of course, male dominated. When the men are sipping scotch after meetings and I'm drinking barley water heavily laced with bicarbonate of soda, I often wonder how they would cope if they had persistent penile infections!

Caroline is 38. She has two teenage children and is separated from her husband. For one reason or another she has suffered from a lot of cystitis over the years.

Cystitis is a problem I always seem to have had. I was a virgin when I got married at 20, but even as a teenager I had a lot of discharge, pain and infection. I think it's a problem that runs in my family. My older sister is always suffering, too, and her daughters have had cystitis and thrush as well.

I've found out from chats with the girls that there's a lot of it about – you know how girls talk when they get together. But when I was younger you couldn't discuss this type of thing at all. Actually, it's quite funny because I remember being a teenager and finding out a bit about venereal disease. There was me, never having had sex in my life, convinced I had VD when it was really just cystitis.

As I said, I was 20 and a virgin when I got married. Sex made me sore and brought on a lot of cystitis. During my second pregnancy I seemed to have cystitis for the whole nine months! I took many courses of antibiotics to try to clear it up, which gave me thrush. As a result, I got so swollen down there that I could hardly walk.

After my son was born, my cystitis eased up a bit. When he was just over two years old, I decided to leave my husband. And since then I've been much better. I'd reached a point when I just couldn't take it any more. It's been hard bringing up two children on my own, but I've learned a lot. I've moved on and I'm stronger now.

I had begun to think 'What the hell is wrong with me? Why am I suffering from cystitis all the time?' It had become normal for me to feel ill! My brother-in-law is a GP and he was very helpful to me – in fact, he really put my mind at ease. He explained that lots of things can trigger the infection, that it wasn't my fault I was suffering. He also suggested that my husband should be treated, too. Often, sexual partners can pass an infection backwards and forwards, reinfecting each other. But my husband was never checked out. I don't think I had the courage to ask him. He never considered that the cystitis was his problem too – it wasn't something that was wrong with him, it was something that was wrong with me. I don't know if my brother-in-law was trying to suggest this to me, but it certainly crossed my mind that my husband might have caught an infection from another woman and passed it on to me. I wouldn't want to accuse him of being unfaithful, but before we split up, there were rumours that he was seeing another woman.

I've only ever had two sexual partners in my life: my husband and my current boyfriend, who I met about a year and a half ago. I'd say he's about 100 per cent more considerate than my husband was. I've only had two attacks since I've been with my new partner and they tend to be triggered by having sex.

When I have an attack, I get a burning pain and terrible backache. I really hate going to the loo when I've got it. Fortunately, I've never had any bleeding, but I get an unpleasant runny, heavy discharge.

In my time, I've been treated by my GP and a special clinic. The doctors there never actually found an infection, although they diagnosed cystitis. I've had a lot of thrush in my time but, touch wood, not for several years. I had my last attack of cystitis two weeks ago. I went to my doctor and took some antibiotics, which cleared it up. In the past, I've treated it myself, though, with Cystemme, which you can buy at the chemist. It tastes like Andrews and seems to help. I also try to drink as much water as possible. I avoid drinking heavily concentrated, acidic juices too. I don't know if this is an old wives' tale, but my Mum always used to say, 'Stay away from hot peppers and spicy foods'. I like curries, but I don't eat them so much anymore.

I always try to pass urine and wash after sex because I've noticed that I get cystitis when I don't. But it's not always convenient to do so. Some partners would be insulted if you got up to have a wash. They might think you were washing all traces of them away!

Kathryn is 30 and suffered cystitis from as far back as she can remember. After years of misdiagnosis from doctors and countless ineffective courses of antibiotics, she eventually sought help from a naturopath. The source of her problem was diagnosed as candida.

Since leaving that first consultation, Kath has followed an anti-candida diet rigorously. She has remained free from cystitis (and colds and other illness you may care to mention) ever since!

I suffered from cystitis for as long as I can remember. My earliest memories are of me sitting on the toilet, crying in agony.

I think I was about four when the problem started, although it was never really identified as cystitis. When I was a child, I was always told I had something wrong with my kidneys. When I went back to school, my excuse note would always say, 'Kathryn is suffering from kidney problems'. But when they did tests, they never found anything wrong with my kidneys.

Every three months I had to go to Great Ormond Street Hospital for tests. I never knew what these were exactly. I remember a tube being stuck up me and having to drink coloured fluids. I would then be X-rayed whilst these worked their way through me. This went on for years and they could never find anything wrong with me. I had a lot of time off school. I also had a lot of antibiotics and eventually I became allergic to almost every kind. Even now I can't take penicillin.

Eventually, when I was about 10 or 11, they took me into hospital. There was some sort of experiment going on there, and I was given an operation to stretch my bladder. It didn't make the problem any better though. Back at school, sometimes the cystitis was so bad I'd have to eat my lunch in the toilet.

When I got to adolescence and started my periods, the cystitis eased off a bit. Between the ages of 13 to 26 I would get about 2 attacks a year. This was manageable compared with almost continuous cystitis I'd suffered with before then – I just sort of coped. My Mum and I experimented to discover the sorts of things that would bring on the symptoms. We found that citrus drinks and fizzy drinks, such as coke or lemonade, were really bad for me. I couldn't eat chocolate, couldn't use bubble baths or any perfumed products and I had to avoid tight jeans. When I reached my late teens, having sex and drinking alcohol became triggers.

When I was 26, I moved to Australia and the attacks began to get more frequent. Eventually, I went to my GP who sent me off to have all the same tests that I'd had as a child. But again, they couldn't find anything wrong. The cystitis attacks continued. Normally I'd go to work and try my best to cope, but one night, when I was on my own in the flat, I had such a bad attack that, at about three o'clock in the morning, I rang a friend and asked her to come over. She took one look at me with my raging fever and took me straight to the hospital. The doctors there were very nice and gave me antibiotics, but I realized then that I couldn't go on like this any more. I just had to do something about the problem myself.

I'd recently got interested in natural medicine, so I contacted a naturopath and made a two-hour appointment with her. For the first time in my life, I felt that someone was actually listening to me. She took down every last detail of my cystitis history, which no doctor had ever done before. She asked me lots of personal questions, which no one had ever asked me before: how was I getting on with my boyfriend, was I breastfed as a child, how many antibiotics did I have as a child? More importantly, no doctor had ever asked me about what I ate. But this woman's cure changed my diet completely.

The naturopath decided that I had candida, which is an overgrowth of yeast throughout the body. She thought the cystitis was just a symptom of this and that the candida problem was caused by the constant supply of antibiotics I was given as a baby. Basically my whole system had been thrown out of balance when I was small and had never recovered. That's why she put me on an anti-candida diet, designed to give my body the perfect environment to get rid of yeasts and restore its natural balance. The naturopath made it clear that I didn't have to go on this diet forever, I just had to give my body time to heal itself.

I was on the diet for six months, although it was very difficult to stick to. I wasn't allowed to have dairy products, caffeine, yeasts or fermented foods – anything that would help yeasts to grow within my body had to be avoided. I wasn't allowed to eat anything that was processed: I had to eat brown rice, brown pasta and yeast-free brown bread. I also couldn't eat any fruit – it's too high in sugar. Papaya and kiwi were allowed because they are low sugar. Going out to a restaurant was difficult because there's always something in every dish that you're not allowed to eat. If I did eat out, I'd always ask for steamed fish with vegetables – that was OK.

I found it really difficult to give up wine, however. Alcohol is usually forbidden but I was allowed a few glasses occasionally, as long as I promised to be strict about everything else. Tea and coffee were hard to give up too. I don't eat meat, so I had to promise the naturopath that I would eat fish at least once a day to keep my protein levels up.

I was also given a whole range of vitamin supplements and herbal potions to take to boost my system. I still take acidophilus every day, although, now I'm back in the UK, it's hard to find shops that stock it. She mixed up a herbal treatment specially for me and I took vitamin C and a multi-vitamin, slippery elm powder, which is a really potent healing powder. For this reason, I think it probably shouldn't be taken in early pregnancy.

For the first few days I had spots, headaches and generally felt disgusting. Everyone at work thought I should stop the diet as it didn't seem to be making me better, but I rang the naturopath who reassured me that what I was feeling was perfectly normal. While my body cleared itself out, I was going to feel rough.

Luckily, my boyfriend was very supportive throughout this time and he made a real effort to find recipes that would fit into my diet. I got completely obsessive about it. I wouldn't eat one mouthful of bread with yeast in it. I think that's the only way to do it actually. After a month, I was very happy about it. I felt so great that the diet didn't seem to be a problem. The good thing about it is that you can eat as much as you like and you don't put on weight because you're only eating foods that are good for your body. Without dairy foods or meat, the diet is very low in fats. I have lots of self-discipline and I was determined to stick to it.

After two weeks, I began to feel really well. I started to exercise and became a total health fanatic. Once you've been through this kind of diet, you notice the difference in your body.

The good news is that I haven't had an attack of cystitis since that first appointment with the naturopath three years ago. After six months on the anti-candida diet I started to eat some of the forbidden foods. And now if I fancy a bit of chocolate cake, I'll have it. But if I go out and end up having a dessert and drinking too much, the next day I feel my body saying, 'Hang on, what do you think you're doing?', so I go back on the diet for a few days and I feel OK again. Being careful about what I eat has put me in control of my cystitis problem and my health. I haven't had a cold in three years. I'll always be very careful about what I eat. Once you've felt *that* good you want to *stay* feeling that good!

Katie is a 24-year-old film editor. Her chronic cystitis in her late teens was cured by having her urethra stretched.

I was 15 when I first got cystitis and I hadn't a clue what was wrong with me. Luckily my Mum knew about cystitis and she explained what it was. She was sympathetic as she'd had cystitis herself, and although she probably realized I'd got it from having sex, she didn't quiz me about it. Both my parents were very anti me having sex, which kind of backfired on them. Their attitude just led me to being completely deceitful to them. I'm not really proud of this because I ended up going out with some pretty horrible men – the types who are only interested in sex and mess you around.

Anyway, I felt this terrible burning pain and I felt like I needed to go to the loo the whole time. I had to go to the doctor immediately, it was really that bad. I've never been certain what caused this first attack. I managed to persuade Mum into thinking I'd got it through wearing tight jeans. It might have been caused by having sex – I'd recently lost my virginity. But it could have been the clothes I used to wear around that time. I used to wear lots of Lycra, tight catsuits, mini-skirts with tights, that sort of thing.

My first bout of cystitis was an isolated attack. My doctor prescribed antibiotics and it cleared up pretty quickly. I had no more problems until about a year later when I started having regular boyfriends and having regular sex. During the next nine months, I had three or four very painful attacks. But then, over the next 18 months I had it almost continuously. When each new bout started up, the pain would be so bad that I couldn't even leave the house, I'd need to go to the loo so often. As the attacks went on, I'd get deeper and deeper infections until, by the time I was 17 and a half, I'd had a couple of kidney infections. It was like having flu every month. I used to feel nauseous and dizzy, and I used to bleed, too.

I had chronic cystitis and I was almost continually on antibiotics. I had pots full of the stuff next to my bed. My doctor also gave me some absolutely foul medicine called mist. pot. cit. I could hardly swallow it, it was so disgusting. To be honest, I never drank it regularly as it was so horrible. Perhaps that's why I got it so much. Actually I don't like drinking anything very much. I'd put bottles of water by my bed and force myself to drink half a bottle before I went to sleep and half a bottle when I woke up. The fact that I hate drinking might have a lot to do with why I got cystitis; my urine must have been very concentrated.

Anyway, my A level examinations were coming up and I think my Mum realized that I couldn't go on like this if I was to have any hope of passing them. We were privately insured at the time and so my Mum took me to my GP to ask for a referral to a cystitis specialist. We got an appointment with a consultant in Harley Street.

First of all, the consultant had to be sure that my kidneys were working properly. So he sent me off for a kidney check where a dye is injected into the bloodstream. Doctors watch a screen that shows the dye travelling round your body and through your kidneys. This proved that they were OK, which made the consultant think the cause of my cystitis must have something to do with my urethra instead. He thought the problem was that I had a very narrow urethra. So, a few months before my A levels, I had an operation, under general anaesthetic, to stretch my urethra. They stick a tube in your urethra all the way to the top, then inflate a sort of balloon which stretches and widens your urethra for good. The theory is that afterwards the urine can flow better which keeps you cystitis-free.

I have heard it said that this operation sometimes makes the problem worse instead of better, but in my case, it was incredible. I had a complete and utter recovery. In the six years since this operation, I've only had it twice and, in each case, I think I know why it recurred.

One of those times happened about four years ago when I was travelling in India. I'd just met the man who was to become my husband and we spent two and a half weeks together, bonking continuously. On our last day together, I got dysentery and cystitis at the same time. That was a nightmare, needing to be sick, wanting to wee and having diarrhoea all at once! I went to a pharmacy and got some strong antibiotics. They didn't cure the dysentery, but they did get rid of the cystitis straight away.

Looking back on those 18 months of cystitis, I don't know how I coped. When it was really bad, I couldn't go anywhere or do anything.

I was very depressed that year, which might have been a reason for my getting ill so often. I was boarding at a school in London and the whole atmosphere was so bad, I spent most of the time in tears. People thought I was a miserable so and so. I don't know how much it was to do with the school, more the people I didn't like! But of course, the cystitis could have been sexually related. At the time I didn't link it with sex – I thought it was something that just kept happening. I can't remember any advice the doctor gave me about sex to avoid cystitis. I had a long-term boyfriend at school who kept ending our relationship only to start it up again soon after. I know now that I was having sex for all the wrong reasons. In fact, I think there were even occasions when I had sex during an attack, but certainly not when it was really bad – I wouldn't have been able to. About a year later I'd left school and started travelling, so I was much happier.

Janine is 44 and a foster mother. She has suffered from years of depression and had many gynaecological operations, including one to reverse her sterilization. A hysterectomy eight years ago left her incontinent. Successive operations on her bladder have meant that she now has cystitis permanently.

I've had a lot of cystitis over the last eight years and I've pretty much got it all the time now. The problem started when I had a hysterectomy. My periods had become so long and so heavy that my gynaecologist thought it best to remove my womb. Initially I felt much better because the bleeding had stopped, but the operation had left me incontinent. If I sneezed, coughed, laughed or ran for the bus I'd wet myself. I couldn't even dance, it was that bad.

I'm not exactly sure what caused this. You have to be careful not to lift anything heavy after a hysterectomy and quite soon afterwards I'd picked up one of the children. At the time I knew I shouldn't have. Anyway, the incontinence gradually got worse until it seemed that I couldn't do anything. Emptying my bladder didn't make any difference – urine still kept leaking out! Eventually, I went to the doctor and said I couldn't stand it any more. I was referred to a urologist at my local hospital, who gave me mild tranquillizers. I took these drugs for two years, but they didn't work, so he decided I ought to have an operation to correct my prolapsed bladder, where the bladder is stitched on either side to pull it back to its proper position. It's a serious operation, done under general anaesthetic, followed by a ten-day stay in hospital.

After the operation, I was still pretty much incontinent. I'd been warned that it might not work and that they might have to repeat it. So a year later, I went under the knife again. It couldn't have happened at a more difficult time. I had a lot of family problems at home. My husband had been accused of hitting one of our foster children. I think the stress was more than I could cope with. The doctors and nurses knew all about the problems I was having at home and were really nice to me. They gave me massages and tried everything to help, but my bladder wouldn't work at all! On the day I left the hospital, my friend picked me up and took me out to lunch. Well, I was sitting in a restaurant and I just wet myself. It wasn't funny at the time, although I can laugh about it now. I went back to the hospital, where they fitted me with a catheter, and I came home.

It was only when the catheter was removed three weeks later, that I realized that this operation had made my problems worse. I wasn't incontinent any more; instead I was unable to empty my bladder! I can drink loads of water yet never manage to pass more than a trickle of urine. A few minutes later, I have to go again because it feels like I haven't been at all. It's like having cystitis all the time, but without the burning pain. And now, to top it all, I actually keep getting cystitis infections, so it does burn and it is painful most of the time! And it's been like this for over three years now.

But, apart from the infections, it's the inconvenience I resent. My friends won't queue for the loo behind me because they know I'll be in there for about ten minutes! The problem is that they've sewn up my bladder too tightly. I've been back to hospital three times to have it stretched, but it hasn't made any difference. The doctors say they can't do it anymore as there's a danger I'll become incontinent again. Where they've sewn it back, there's a ridge of scar tissue, so if I have intercourse – which is very rarely these days – it's very painful. I'm going to have an operation to get rid of the scar tissue soon. This should mean that my bladder is able to empty itself fully once again. And hopefully, this will see an end to the cystitis attacks.

The last time I had an attack, it took me a week to go to my GP. I'm fed up with seeing her. I feel as though I spend my life at the surgery. The antibiotics I'm prescribed don't seem to work, they simply give me thrush. This then triggers another attack of cystitis – it's a vicious circle; I've had two lots of antibiotics in three weeks! To stop the burning, my GP gave me Effercitrate tablets. These dissolve in water and make your urine less acidic. They're quite effective. I'm supposed to take them when I feel the cystitis coming on. Perhaps I should take them all the time!

At one stage, the specialists thought I should try using a catheter three times a day to empty my bladder myself. It might help, but I know that using a catheter can cause infections.

I just want something to work. I get so depressed about it. They say that stress makes it worse. That's probably why I've got it continually, because I'm stressed all the time. Looking back on the last eight years, I wouldn't recommend any woman to have a hysterectomy. It's been the cause of so many other problems.

Ruth is 72. She has had cystitis several times during the last 50 years, but over the years, she has learnt to cope and prevent further attacks starting.

My doctor used to pooh-pooh the idea that getting one's feet soaking wet could cause a bout of cystitis. He thought this was just an old wives' tale, but it happened to me – twice. Perhaps it was just a coincidence? I had been watering the garden when the hose burst and completely soaked me from the knees downwards. I'm 72, but I can remember my Grandmother suffering from the same thing. In our family it was just accepted that if you got your feet wet you'd get cystitis.

I had my first attack when I was a young woman of 23. I'd started sleeping with my boyfriend, who later became my husband. We used to go into the fields and spend the night there together. When I got my first attack of cystitis, I put it down to the fact that I'd been lying on wet grass. No way did I put it down to what we'd been doing. It was only years later, after reading a book on cystitis, that I realized it was linked with sexual activity.

Actually, the first time I got cystitis it scared the living daylights out of me. Since then I've had far worse attacks – if I remember correctly this one was quite slight. Anyway, I trotted round to my doctor's, who put me in hospital – yes, really!

It was 1945, and I spent eight weeks in hospital. I nearly lost my job at the time – my boss wanted to know what it was that was keeping me in there so long. Looking back on it now I think I was used as a bit of a guinea pig. But you know what it's like when you're young, you tend to put yourself in doctors' hands and not question their actions. I had to stay in bed – despite the fact that I felt perfectly all right – while they carried out a big investigation as to what could have caused it. Now I know what the culprit was – it happened after just one night of sex! But no one ever asked me about this or put two and two together.

I had to have an intravenous pyelography, a most unpleasant experience in those days. I had to lie on a cold slab, the X-ray table, whilst dye injected into a vein was photographed as it passed through the blood vessels into my kidneys and into my bladder. I remember having a catheter inserted too, which was most painful and made me very sore, whereas I hadn't been before. They couldn't find anything wrong and eventually, after two months, I was allowed to go home. I think the cystitis had cleared up of it's own accord not long after it had started!

Years later I had another bout of cystitis – a very bad one. I had an important job at the time, but I left work and belted up to the surgery to find a huge queue for the doctor. I was hopping about from one leg to the other in the waiting room and the doctor saw me and told me he'd see me straight away. I had antibiotics to clear it up this time, but I remember having another attack shortly after this. So I went back to the surgery and saw Dr B instead of my usual Dr A. He sent me to hospital again to see a specialist. He investigated the problem, but couldn't find anything wrong with me. I admitted to him that I hadn't thought anything was wrong either, but that my doctor had made me come. Apparently the specialist then gave poor old Dr B a right rollicking for sending me there in the first place. Later I told my own doctor the story. I'll always remember his reply: 'Good gracious,' he said, 'if I sent every woman to hospital who came into this surgery with cystitis I'd be out of business.' So it must be rife, mustn't it?

Gill is 42 with three children and has suffered from chronic cystitis for the last seven years. No infection has ever been found, although she has been prescribed heaps of antibiotics since then. She is still

exploring possible causes of the problem and is struggling to cope emotionally.

I've had cystitis for so long now, I know the locations of practically every loo in south east England.

After my second child was born in 1982, I had acute attacks of cystitis. The doctors never found an infection present. But even so, they would prescribe antibiotics as a treatment. The attacks did clear up, although I was sometimes left with low-level symptoms. But I remember having long periods without any cystitis at all until my son was born in 1985. Then, when he was about four months old, I started suffering again, and I've suffered ever since.

I have this constant desire to pass water. I go to the loo, then I find I have to go five minutes later. I'm always aware of my bladder, nagging away at me. The feeling like I need to urinate is always there. I just have to ignore it. Sometimes this is easy, sometimes it's really hard. It's debilitating and depressing and affects my whole life.

I can't take my classes on school trips – I'm a geography teacher. Luckily, I've taught at the same school for 19 years and they've been very good about it. But while I'm suffering from this cystitis, I can't think about changing jobs.

With the acute attacks I'd initially experienced, I'd been treated by my GP and investigated by a urologist. Eventually I made an appointment with a private urologist who, unfortunately, was no help whatsoever. Then I went to see a private cystitis counsellor, who was great! She spent two hours with me, which went like ten minutes. She gave me about 15 things to work through that could ease the problem, ranging from going to the loo immediately after sex down to taking mineral supplements and having an allergy test. I worked my way through this list, but nothing seemed to make a difference. The counsellor's understanding and support, however, helped me more than any of the practical advice she was to give me.

Over the last seven years, I've tried many alternative therapies. When I was very low, I went to an acupuncturist. The baby was still very small and things were really grim. I went three times a week, but eventually, I realized that I wasn't getting anywhere. I think if acupuncture was going to work *my* acupuncturist would have cured me. She was very good, an extremely caring no-nonsense type of woman. It was a tonic just to be treated by somebody like that. I think her personality was more helpful than her treatments. I felt supported by that woman; she even gave me six or seven treatments for free.

I've seen a homeopath, an osteopath and a herbalist. I wasn't impressed at all by the herbalist – he seemed to be too quick to decide what the matter was. He gave me some awful pills, which made the cystitis much much worse. I persevered for about three days and then gave up. They were driving me round the bend. My husband always said I should have continued with them. He thinks if I had that they might have worked.

My husband has been brilliant, really super. He's had to put up with a lot. For 18 months, we didn't have penetrative sex at all. Then I came to my senses and realized that not having sex wasn't making any difference – I still had cystitis.

For the last nine months, I've been going privately to see a psychologist. We haven't made much progress. She believes that people's problems arise when they are very young, that the root cause of my cystitis might be a childhood incident which hasn't been resolved yet. So together, we've been going over my past. I wish I could find something there, but I had a very conventional, happy childhood. So if *this* caused a problem, then God help everybody else who wasn't so lucky.

I know I'm not imagining my problem because I recently had a cystoscopy, which revealed large areas of my bladder to be inflamed and sore. I have wondered if I might have interstitial cystitis and I've read Dr Larrian Gillespie's book on the matter. The symptoms she described seemed different to mine, but I thought I'd try her self-help plan anyway. I followed her dietary advice and took the recommended vitamin supplements. I can't say it really helped though.

The only thing that alleviates my symptoms is hard physical exercise, which I try to do two or three times a week. Sometimes I feel lousy, but I make myself play badminton and I can feel the difference. It's not just that sport takes my mind of the cystitis, it actually improves the symptoms.

Having cystitis has completely ruined my life. The worst thing about it is that I feel so helpless; there doesn't seem to be anything I can do about it. I can just about put up with the pain, but I resent the fact that I have to put so much energy into coping with it.

I try to find something positive about my suffering and accept it. I think because I've got this maybe I won't get some of the more serious diseases in life.

17

Getting to the root of the problem

Use the at-a-glance diagnosis chart in this chapter as your cause and cure checklist. It lists all the possible causes of cystitis and what you can do to help yourself and prevent recurrent attacks.

Anyone suffering from frequent attacks should sit down and go through every aspect of their life with a fine toothcomb. Somewhere there will be an explanation as to why the infection hasn't cleared in the first place or keeps recurring.

But it's important to remember that there may be more than *one* cause underlying any particular attack. That's why it's worth reading the whole book, even sections that you may not think are relevant. With the help of this chart and the rest of the book you should get to the root of your problem.

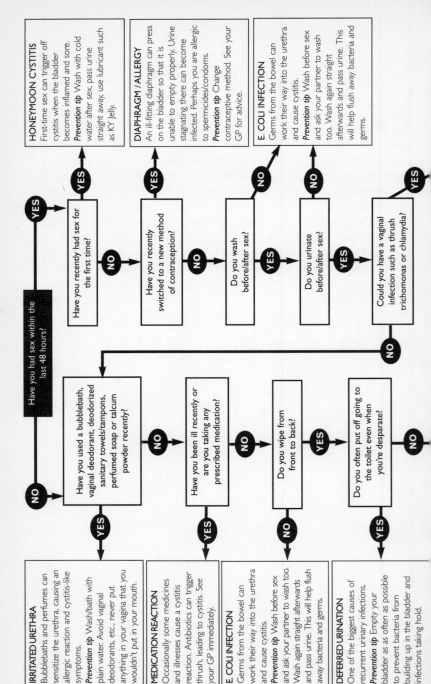

Have you had sex within the last 48 hours?

YES → Have you recently had sex for the first time?

NO → Have you used a bubblebath, vaginal deodorant, deodorized sanitary towels/tampons, perfumed soap or talcum powder recently?

HONEYMOON CYSTITIS
First-time sex can trigger off cystitis when the bladder becomes inflamed and sore. *Prevention tip* Wash with cold water after sex, pass urine straight away, use lubricant such as KY Jelly.

Have you recently had sex for the first time? **NO** → Have you recently switched to a new method of contraception?

YES → **DIAPHRAGM / ALLERGY**
An ill-fitting diaphram can press on the bladder so that it is unable to empty properly. Urine stagnating there can become infected. Perhaps you are allergic to spermicides/condoms. *Prevention tip* Change contraceptive method. See your GP for advice.

Have you recently switched to a new method of contraception? **NO** → Do you wash before/after sex?

Do you wash before/after sex? **NO** → **E. COLI INFECTION**
Germs from the bowel can work their way into the urethra and cause cystitis. *Prevention tip* Wash before sex and ask your partner to wash too. Wash again straight afterwards and pass urine. This will help flush away bacteria and germs.

Do you wash before/after sex? **YES** → Do you urinate before/after sex?

Do you urinate before/after sex? **NO** → **E. COLI INFECTION**

Do you urinate before/after sex? **YES** → Could you have a vaginal infection such as thrush trichomonas or chlamydia?

Could you have a vaginal infection such as thrush trichomonas or chlamydia? **YES** →

Could you have a vaginal infection such as thrush trichomonas or chlamydia? **NO** →

IRRITATED URETHRA
Bubblebaths and perfumes can sensitize the urethra, causing an allergic reaction and cystitis-like symptoms. *Prevention tip* Wash/bath with plain water. Avoid vaginal deodorants, etc., never put anything in your vagina that you wouldn't put in your mouth.

Have you used a bubblebath, vaginal deodorant, deodorized sanitary towels/tampons, perfumed soap or talcum powder recently? **YES** → (IRRITATED URETHRA)

NO → Have you been ill recently or are you taking any prescribed medication?

MEDICATION REACTION
Occasionally some medicines and illnesses cause a cystitis reaction. Antibiotics can trigger thrush, leading to cystitis. See your GP immediately.

Have you been ill recently or are you taking any prescribed medication? **YES** → (MEDICATION REACTION)

NO → Do you wipe from front to back?

E. COLI INFECTION
Germs from the bowel can work their way into the urethra and cause cystitis. *Prevention tip* Wash before sex and ask your partner to wash too. Wash again straight afterwards and pass urine. This will help flush away bacteria and germs.

Do you wipe from front to back? **NO** → (E. COLI INFECTION)

YES → Do you often put off going to the toilet even when you're desparate?

DEFERRED URINATION
One of the biggest causes of recurrent urinary infections. *Prevention tip* Empty your bladder as often as possible to prevent bacteria from building up in the bladder and infections taking hold.

Do you often put off going to the toilet even when you're desparate? **YES** → (DEFERRED URINATION)

NO →

VAGINAL INFECTIONS

Bacteria present in infective vaginal discharge can irritate the urethra. The more profuse the discharge, the more severe and painful this irritation will be. Both thrush and trichomonas can arise naturally in the body. They may also be acquired from your sexual partner. Other more serious sexually-transmitted infections, such as chlamydia, can cause cystitis-like symptoms and need accurate diagnosis and treatment. *Prevention tip* Practise safe sex. Keep the vagina acid to avoid thrush and gardnerella infections taking hold.

ANXIETY/UNEXPLAINED ATTACKS

Emotional ill-health can cause physical pain. The emotions are closely linked with the bladder. Counselling, self-help remedies and/or alternative therapies might offer a cure.

CASE NEEDS FURTHER DIAGNOSIS

Anatomical abnormalities, such as kidney stones and fibroids, can cause cystitis-like symptoms. Ask your GP to refer you to a urologist for further tests.

Do you wear tights, or tight trousers a lot?

NO → **Have you recently had a baby?**

NO → **Have you changed your diet recently?**

NO → **Have you just had a period?**

NO → **Have you suffered from repeated unexplained attacks of cystitis and taken antibiotics for them in the past?**

NO → **Have you been depressed or anxious recently?**

NO → CASE NEEDS FURTHER DIAGNOSIS

YES → ANXIETY/UNEXPLAINED ATTACKS

YES → INTERSTITIAL CYSTITIS

INTERSTITIAL CYSTITIS

This is a non-bacterial inflammation of the bladder, sharing similar symptoms to cystitis. This condition is often caused by taking antibiotics in the absence of bacterial infection. See your GP.

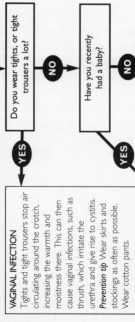

VAGINAL INFECTION

Tights and tight trousers stop air circulating around the crotch, increasing the warmth and moistness there. This can then cause vaginal infections, such as thrush, which irritate the urethra and give rise to cystitis. *Prevention tip* Wear skirts and stockings as often as possible. Wear cotton pants.

WEAKENED MUSCLES/PROLAPSED WOMB

Even a slightly prolapsed womb may be pressing on your bladder so that it is unable to empty properly. Urine allowed to stagnate in the bladder can easily become infected. *Prevention tip* Improve pelvic muscle tone with special pelvic floor exercises.

DIET

Certain foods can trigger cystitis. If you've changed your diet recently, look at your eating to see which food could be the culprit. *Prevention tip* Avoid sugary, sweet foods. Avoid tea, coffee and alcohol. These are diuretics which make you want to pass water.

SANITARY PROTECTION

Using tampons can cause cystitis. The chemicals in super-absorbant/deodorized sanitary towels and tampons can irritate and inflame the vagina and urethra. *Prevention tip* Avoid tampons. Never use deodorized towels. Change towels regularly.

Notes

Kiku Adatto, MA, Kathleen Gormale Doebele, RN, MSW, Leo Galland, MD, Linda Granowetter, MD, 'Behavioural factors and urinary tract infection', *JAMA*, vol. 241, no. 23 (8 June 1979).

C. E. Cox and F. Hinman, Jr, 'Experiments with induced bacterium, vesical emptying and bacterial growth on the mechanism of bladder defense to infection', *Journal of Urology*, vol. 86 (1962), pp. 739–48.

J. Fowler and T. A. Stamey, 'Studies of introital colonization in women with recurrent urinary infections', VII, 'The role of bacterial adherence', *Journal of Urology*, vol. 117 (1977), pp. 472–6.

Aino Jonasson, Bertil Larrson and Helmut Pschera, 'Testing and training of the pelvic floor muscles after childbirth', *Acta Obstet Gynecol Scand*, vol. 68 (1989), pp. 301–4.

M. G. Le et al. 'Alcoholic Beverage Consumption and Breast Cancer in a French Care-Control Study', *American Journal of Epidemiology*, vol. 244, no. 3 (September 1986) pp. 244–7.

M. R. Miles, L. Olson and A. Rogers, 'Recurrent Vaginal Candidiasis: The importance of an intestinal reservoir', *JAMA*, Vol. 234, (1977), pp. 1836–83.

D. V. Moen, 'Observations on the Effectiveness of Cranberry Juice in Urinary Infections', *Wisconsin Medical Journal*, vol. 61, pp. 282–3.

P. Norton and J. Baker, 'Randomised prospective trial of vaginal cones vs Kegel exercises in postpartum primiparous women', Proceedings of the International Continence Society, *Neurology and Urodynamics*, vol. 9, no. 4 (September 1990).

A. B. Peattie, S. Plevnik and S. Stanton, 'Vaginal cones: a conservative method of treating genuine stress incontinence', *British Journal of Obstetrics and Gynaecology*, vol. 95 (October 1988), pp. 1049–53.

The Practitioner, vol. 227 (May 1983), pp. 833–5.

Useful addresses

Allergy information

Action Against Allergy (AAA)
PO Box 278
Middlesex TW1 4QQ

British Allergy Foundation
Deepdene House
30 Bellegrove Road
Welling, Kent DA16 3DY
Tel: 020-8303 8792

The British Society for Allergy and Environmental Medicine
PO Box 28
Totton
Southampton SO30 2ZA

Breakspear Hospital for Allergy and Environmental Medicine
Belswains Lane
Hemel Hempstead
Hertfordshire HP3 9HP
Tel: 01442 61333

Research and general information

The Women's Health Information Centre
52 Featherstone Street
London EC1Y 8RT
Tel: 020-7251 6580
(Open Monday, Wednesday, Thursday and Friday between 10 am and 4 pm)

Professional bodies for practitioners of complementary medicine

The Institute for Complementary Medicine
PO Box 94
London SE16 7QZ
Tel: 020-7237 5165

Register of the Society of Homeopaths
2 Artizan Road
Northampton NN1 4HU
Tel: 01604 621400

National Institute of Medical Herbalists
56 Longbrook Street
Exeter
Devon EX4 6AH
Tel: 01392 426022

Osteopathic Information Service
Osteopathy House
176 Tower Bridge Road
London SE1 3LU
Tel: 020-7357 6655

The International Federation of Aromatherapists
182 Chiswick High Road
London W4 1PP
Tel: 020-8742 2605

British School of Reflexology
The Holistic Healing Centre
92 Sheering Road
Old Harlow
Essex CM17 0JW
Tel: 02179 429060

British Acupuncture Council
63 Jeddo Road
London W12 9HQ
Tel: 020-8735 0400

Homeopathic medicines by mail order

Ainsworth's Pharmacy
38 New Cavendish Street
London W1M 7LH
Tel: 020-7935 5330

Goulds Chemists
14 Crowndale Road
London NW1 1TT
Tel: 020-7388 4752

Helios Homeopathic Pharmacy
97 Camden Road
Tunbridge Wells
Kent TN1 2QR
Tel: 01892 536393

A. Nelson & Co. Limited
73 Duke Street
London W1M 6BY
Tel: 020-7629 3118

Weleda UK Limited
Heanor Road
Ilkeston
Derbyshire DE7 8DR
Tel: 0115 9309319

Cranberry juice capsules

The Nutricentre
7 Park Crescent
London W1N 3HE
Tel: 020-7436 5122

Tea Tree oil treatments

House of Mistry
15–17 Southend Road
Hampstead
London
Tel: 020-7794 0848

Potter's Antitis herbal cystitis tablets

Potter's (Herbal Supplies) Limited
Leyland Mill Lane
Wigan WN1 2SB
Tel: 01942 34761

AIDS

National AIDS helpline: 0800 567123

Non-latex condoms

Schmid Laboratories
PO Box 2337
Anderson
South Carolina
USA

Femina Cones by mail order

Colgate Medical Limited
Shirley Avenue
Windsor
Berkshire SL4 5LH
Tel: 01753 860378 *Fax*: 01753 831137

One-legged tights by mail order

Innovations (Mail Order) Limited
Euroway Business Park
Swindon SN5 8SN
Tel: 01793 514666

Index